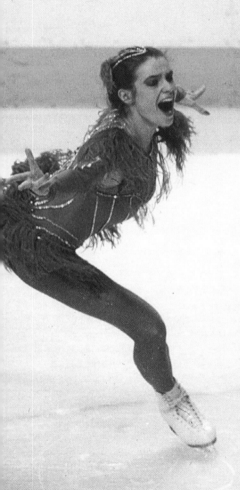

Also available at all good book stores

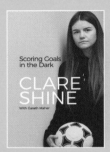

9781801501170

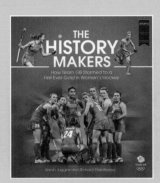

9781785313301

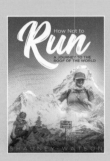

9781785314537

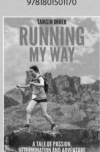

9781785314544

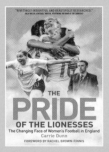

9781785315411

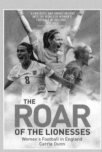

9781785311512

SYNTHETIC MEDALS

Joseph Tudor

SYNTHETIC MEDALS

East German Athletes' Journey to Hell

First published by Pitch Publishing, 2022

Pitch Publishing
9 Donnington Park,
85 Birdham Road,
Chichester,
West Sussex,
PO20 7AJ
www.pitchpublishing.co.uk
info@pitchpublishing.co.uk

ISBN 978 1 80150 135 4

Typesetting and origination by Pitch Publishing
Printed and bound in India by Replika Press Pvt. Ltd.

CONTENTS

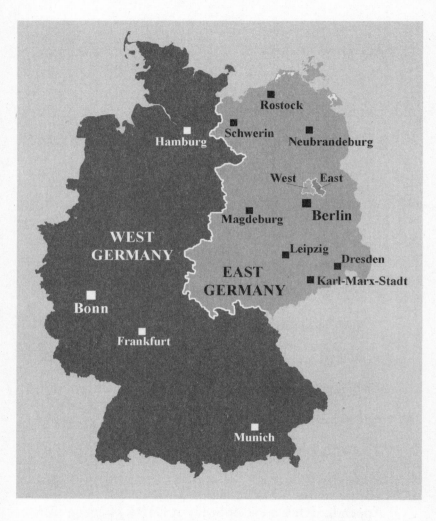

Map of the two Germanys in the period 1949–1990

ACKNOWLEDGEMENTS

FIRST AND foremost, I would like to express my thanks to **Dr Steven Ungerleider**, psychologist and member of the International Paralympic Committee, for his generous access to his bestselling book *Faust's Gold* (St Martin's Press) and subsequent film *Doping for Gold* (BBC/PBS) and additional archival materials on the East German doping protocols.

The production of this book has been possible thanks to the support of some amazing people that have contributed to its final form with their professional input.

Josie, my wonderful other half, whose medical and linguistic knowledge has been of the utmost importance for me to fully understand certain physiological mechanisms of the human body and some German expressions. Her childhood spent in Hamburg has proven to be very useful.

Martin, my son, for his help, encouragement and support.

Silke McNair-Wilson, teacher of German and friend, for helping me translate some complex sentences.

Brenda Ellis, guiding light, for her precious advice regarding the nuances of the English language.

John Paul Kleiner, for granting me access to some very relevant information and pictures from his outstanding website, GDR Objectified, a really fine source of all sorts of materials related to the history of East Germany.

Honourable mentions also go to **Renata Bertola**, with whom I often share my writing experience, and **Claudio Secco** and **Davide Angelini** for their special support.

Special thanks go to:

Dr Daniela Richter, psychology consultant to the LAMV centre in Schwerin (Germany), for her patience in explaining in great detail her incredible job with former GDR athletes in the state of Mecklenburg-Vorpommern.

Dr Sigurd Hanke, chief surgeon at the Delitzsch and Eilenburg clinics (Leipzig), former SC Turbine Erfurt and GDR swimmer, for sharing his life experience as an athlete and as an East German citizen, and for his precious comments and advice.

Last, but not least, all my thanks go to **Dr Ines Geipel**, former SC Motor Jena and GDR sprinter, for her kindness in answering some questions and for showing me the work of her organisation, Doping-Opfer-Hilfe.

INTRODUCTION

THE AIM of this book is to provide all sports fans and contemporary history buffs with a solid and up-to-date reference on one of the most controversial phenomena of the 20th century: state-sponsored doping in East Germany during the Cold War years.

News reports often tell stories of drug scandals which cast a long shadow over the moral integrity of sportsmen and sportswomen. Too often we have seen sprinters, cyclists, swimmers, and competitors of all sorts, trying to cut corners and reach for glory with the help of 'specialist centres' able to supply the athletes with wondrous pharmaceutical supports. Such shortcuts have proven to be both illegal and dangerous.

In the case of the East German athletes, however, there was a major difference: the state itself was the architect of a complex system of secret research, experimentation and distribution of drugs which were surreptitiously administered to the competitors. Most athletes, especially the youngest, didn't have a choice; they got caught, sadly, in a sort of chemical whirlwind of amazing tablets and injections that made them run faster, jump longer and recover from fatigue more effectively, and, in some cases, made them live a shorter life.

The gossip about the doped East German superhumans, and especially about those 'masculine' women, who managed to push a small European country to the top of the medal tables in a variety of sports events, had been circulating for years. It was a topic of discussion among pundits and commentators of all nations. After the fall of the Berlin Wall, and the subsequent collapse of the German Democratic Republic, the truth came out: the East Germans won so much because they cheated. News of confessions and investigations reached the rest of the world, but most of the information and historical analysis about this incredible state-sponsored doping case has remained restricted to the German media.

In English, there are only two relevant works on the topic: one 'popular', the ground-breaking Steven Ungerleider's *Faust's Gold* (St Martin's Press, 2013), and the other 'academic', the excellent Mike Dennis and Jonathan Grix's *Sport Under Communism – Behind the East German Miracle* (Palgrave Macmillan, 2012). The book you are holding is the third; its aim is to tell the story without neglecting a little historical analysis.

Although some of the information you are about to read relies necessarily on the two works above, the vast majority of the material presented here is based on recent information collected through interviews that various athletes and other protagonists have given, mainly to the German press; I have had the chance to personally talk to some of them. This is therefore a book that aims to bring together the most up-to-date revelations, sorting them into themes, in order to provide a better understanding of the state-sponsored doping phenomenon. There are so many personal stories that deserve to be told; I thought it was only right to make them available to a wider public.

Furthermore, I have attempted to analyse the rise of the GDR in the context of the post-Second World War years and the Cold War period, and try to evaluate the reasons that piloted its political leaders in developing and implementing the notorious plan that sold the soul of its children to the devil.

The story narrated in this book can be seen as a thriller, complete with victims, spies, conspirators, shadowy characters and heroes, races against time and plot twists. It's a long story that tells of fake and real victories, of pain and atonement. The story even bears a supernatural element: a demonic pact between the East German government and an evil entity disguised in white lab coats. I will also explore the consequences of that deal, generated by the distorted achievements of modern chemistry, the real Philosopher's Stone of the 20th century, able to change the ambitions of an unscrupulous state leadership into gold.

In the first three chapters we'll explore the circumstances that enabled the investigators to discover the state-sponsored doping system, and how political leaders and scientists created it. We'll try to analyse the historical reasons that pushed the GDR government to develop a very well organised network which was perfectly integrated within an extraordinary scheme of recruitment and training of athletes.

In chapters four and five we'll have a look at the *Dopingprozess*, the trial that showed the world the state-sponsored doping system thanks to the confessions of athletes, managers and political leaders. Here, we can read the harsh testimonies of several protagonists of the East German regime, which will help us to understand the reasons for their decisions and the relative consequences on the athletes' lives.

In chapters six, seven and eight, different aspects related to drug use in sport will be examined, including a glance into the difficult lives of the former athletes and how they have been coping with their health after the end of their career, and the hypocrisy that often surrounds the world of sport. Also, some brief analysis of the political, social and economic background of the years 1945–89 will help us understand the development of the 'pharmaceutical connection' in that period.

Finally, in the last chapter, we delve into the means of social support, both financial and moral, that the newly united Germany decided to offer to the victims of the GDR state-sponsored doping programme.

The path through the pages of this book will not be easy: it is a disturbing journey into a tainted aspect of the human soul. The main intention is to inform the readers, while trying to instil in them the curiosity to explore more about a topic which certainly deserved a greater degree of attention from the media.

Joseph Tudor

LIST OF ACRONYMS

ASK   *Armeesportklub* (Military Sports Club)
BA   *Bundesarchiv* (Federal Archive)
BFC   *Berliner Fussballclub Dynamo* (Dynamo Berlin FC)
BStU   *Bundesbeauftragte für die Unterlagen des Staatssicherheitsdienstes der ehemaligen Deutschen Demokratischen Republik* (Federal Commissioner for the Records of the Security Service of the former German Democratic Republic)
DDR   *Deutschen Demokratischen Republik* (GDR, German Democratic Republic)
DHfK   *Deutsche Hochschule für Körperkultur* (German University for Physical Education)
DOSB   *Der Deutsche Olympische Sportbund* (German Olympic Sports Federation)
DSV   *Deutscher Fußball Verband* (German Football Association)
DSSV   *Deutsche Schwimmsport-Verband* (German Swimming Association)
DTSB   *Deutscher Turn und Sportbund* (German Gymnastics and Sports Federation)
ESA   *Einheitiliche Sichtung und Auswahl* (Uniform Sifting and Selection)
FDJ   *Freie Deutsche Jugend* (Free German Youth)
FIFA   *Fédération Internationale de Football Association*
FINA   *Fédération Internationale de Natation* (International Swimming Federation)
FKS   *Forschungsinstitut für Körperkultur und Sport* (Research Institute for Physical Culture and Sport)
FRG   *Federal Republic of Germany* (West Germany)
IAAF   *International Associations of Athletics Federations*
IM   *Inoffizielle Mitarbeiter* (Unofficial Collaborator)
IOC   International Olympic Committee

KJS	*Kinder und Jugendsportschulen* (Children and Youth's Sports Schools)
LAMV	*Landesbeauftragten für Mecklenburg-Vorpommern für die Aufarbeitung der SED-Diktatur* (State representative for Mecklenburg-Vorpommern for Coming to Terms with the SED Dictatorship)
NOC	*Nationales Olympisches Komitee der DDR (National Olympic Committee of the German Democratic Republic)*
SC	*Sport Club* (a special boarding school where children could study and practise sport)
SED	*Sozialistische Einheitspartei Deutschlands* (Socialist Unity Party of Germany)
SKS	*Staatssekretariat für Körperkultur und Sport* (State Committee for Physical Culture and Sport)
SMD	*Sportmedizinischer Dienst der DDR* (Sports Medical Service of the GDR)
STASI	*Staatssicherheit* (Ministry for State Security)
TZ	*Trainings-Zentren* (Training Centre)
UEFA	*Union of European Football Associations*
UM	*Unterstützende Mittel* (Supportive Means)
USA	United States of America
USSR	Union of Soviet Socialist Republics (Soviet Union)
VEB	*Volkseigener Betrieb* (Publicly Owned Enterprise)
ZA	*Zentralarchiv* (Central Archive)
ZERV	*Zentrale Ermittlungsstelle für Regierungs und Vereinigungskriminalität* (Central Investigation Agency for Government and Association Crime)
ZI	*Zentralinstitut* (Central Institute – laboratory in Kreischa, near Dresden)
ZIMET	*Zentralinstitut für Mikrobiologie und experimentelle Therapie* (Central Institute for Microbiology and Experimental Therapy)

1

DIE WENDE: BEFORE AND
AFTER THE WALL

ON 9 November 1989, the Berlin Wall, symbol of the ideological and geographical separation between West Germany and East Germany and, by extension, between Western Europe and Eastern Europe, is finally knocked down after 28 years. Among millions of cheering Germans celebrating their newly acquired freedom – perhaps while listening to an improvised solo concert by the Russian cellist Rostropovich on top of concrete rubble and dusty bricks – a few people are incessantly busy, destroying piles of compromising documents: several thousand folders containing secret files and classified records efficiently collected and religiously collated in the last 40 years by the *Ministerium für Staatsicherheit*, the notorious secret police agency also known as the *Stasi*, which operated in the German Democratic Republic between 1950 and 1990. Priority is given to documents containing the names of spies, informers and undercover agents. In a few days, tons of papers are reduced to confetti by shredding machines; very soon, the pavements around the *Ministerium* building on Ruschestraße begin to look like the streets of Rio de Janeiro after the Carnival.

After the Second World War, Germany had been divided by the Allies into two different countries: West Germany came under the influence of the western powers (USA, UK and France), whilst East Germany was essentially controlled by the Soviet Union. The two states had evolved along diverging paths: the former a capitalist/democratic nation, the latter a communist/totalitarian regime. The German Democratic Republic had many dark secrets but by 1989 it has collapsed. It's clear to everyone that its entire political and bureaucratic structure is about to disintegrate, and buried secrets are going to emerge, creating a lot of trouble for those who have governed the country until then.

One of the most efficient (and disturbing) aspects of the GDR was its colossal spying system – cleverly organised as a pyramidal structure – which was totally dedicated to the surveillance of its citizens. The sudden fall of the country means that from the steel cabinets hosted in the main building of the *Stasi*, in Berlin, could soon emerge scandals that the German officials would certainly like to avoid.

They only partially succeed, as the East German citizens (and the whole world) eventually find out about that shocking system and, above all, the disquieting fact that even relatives and friends had spied on each other for many years, faithfully annotating secrets, gossip and information of various origins and reporting them to the Ministry officers. Despite the intent to destroy everything, many documents survive thanks to the immense extent of the *Stasi* archive; ironically, the huge number of documents collected in nearly 40 years of secret surveillance made its total elimination very difficult.

East German citizens are soon pushing to get access to those archives. In December 1991, the government of united Germany passes the *Stasi-Unterlagen-Gesetz*, a type of freedom of information act to guarantee access for all people to the Ministry of State Security's archives which survived the purge. The sudden political and social changes related to the post-Wall period (branded by the Germans as *Die Wende*), and the awareness of living unexpectedly in a democratic and liberal state, persuades millions of East German citizens to consult the *Stasi* archives to check if there was a secret folder about them – many found out that there was (at least) one! The discovery of the incredible number of crimes contained in those files sparks so much indignation that in 1991 the German parliament launches the ZERV[1], a government agency to investigate the most serious offences committed during the years of the regime, led by Walter Ulbricht (1950–71) and Erich Honecker (1971–89). Nearly 300 detectives, commanded by Manfred Kittlaus, look into crimes of various levels against the people of East Germany. A very evocative illustration of the oppressive control suffered by these citizens can be appreciated in the Academy Award and BAFTA-winning film *Lives of the Others* (Florian Henckel von Donnersmarck, 2006).

Many crimes are investigated but a few years later, in 2000, the ZERV is disbanded, as its promoters realise that the majority of the offences, which relate to human rights violations, are very difficult to prove. Besides, many of the perpetrators would never spend a day in prison because of the statute of limitations. In order to avoid a waste of public money, and also to spare anyone's embarrassment, it is decided to close for good that particular chapter of East Germany's history.

When all seems lost and justice denied, an incredible discovery gives a decisive boost of hope; as we'll see, in time, several transgressions eventually emerge from oblivion and are dealt with accordingly.

Brigitte and Werner

Among the various documents in the *Stasi* archives, in the 'Sport' section ('Department XX/3'), there were papers related to one of the best-guarded secrets in the country: a state-sponsored plan for the research and use of doping, tested on

---

1   Central Investigative Agency for Government and Organised Crime (*Zentrale Ermittlungsstelle für Regierungs und Vereinigungskriminalität*).

and administered to GDR athletes, very often without their consent or knowledge. Obviously, diligent officers of the *Ministerium* tried (and, to some extent, succeeded) to destroy all files connected to that hideous system; the sudden wave of democratic freedom, due to the reunification of the two Germanys, might have pushed former athletes, or even curious researchers, to look for evidence regarding the unconventional 'training practices' that took place within the walls of the various sports clubs. It was highly advisable to make those documents disappear.

However, a couple of researchers took an interest in those files and tried to prevent their obliteration: former athlete Brigitte Berendonk and her husband, biologist Werner Franke.

During the Olympics in Mexico City, in 1968, young Brigitte is resting on a semi-rusted bench inside the locker room of the *Estadio Universitario*. Her thoughts are mainly devoted to the discus throw final that is about to start; she is one of the finalists and she will try to achieve the best result possible for herself and her country, West Germany. Next to her, three East German athletes, Anita Otto, Christine Spielberg and Karen Illgen, improvise warming-up routines in the narrow spaces available. Brigitte observes them and can't help wondering if those athletes have qualified on merit and without taking drugs.[2] Brigitte asks herself such a question because she is a former GDR athlete who defected to West Germany a few years earlier and knows that in East Germany there have been significant studies into the use of doping – she is seriously speculating on the fairness of the competition ahead. She will come eighth but the GDR trio will also finish out of the medals and none have ever been linked to the doping programme.[3]

---

2   Steven Ungerleider, *Faust's Gold*, St Martin's Press, 2013.

3   The best performer among the GDR athletes was Anita Otto, who finished fourth.

In many interviews, Berendonk has told her personal story, especially highlighting the years of adolescence in a pre-Wall East Germany; she often remarks that after completing compulsory school, at 14, children who wished to carry on with their studies had to belong to a family with strong connections with the political world. Given her good sporting skills, and her dad being a renowned doctor, young Brigitte managed to get an offer at a prestigious sports club in Leipzig: 'They asked me what would I like to do after my sports career ... they wanted to assure us that the state would take care of us ... they were very seductive. But if I didn't have athletic skills, then I would be sent back home.'[4] It looked like blackmail. The state would take care of all the students' needs but it wanted super-human beings in exchange. Although it wasn't clear at that time, Brigitte Berendonk is now convinced she attended a 'friendly prison' rather than a school and recalls a sense of being part of a big experiment. The drugs weren't fully developed yet but Dr Berendonk (her father) knew that certain substances were beginning to circulate among the athletes. He also knew enough about the level of corruption and oppression that was developing in his country and at some point, he realised he didn't want his family to live in such a hostile environment. He decided to leave Eisenach, their home town, and took his wife and children across the border to West Berlin.

Brigitte Berendonk then grew up as an athlete in West Germany, aware of the obscure practices taking place on the other side of the *Berliner Mauer*. Soon after the Olympic Games in Mexico and even more so after Munich (1972), she began to boldly denounce certain GDR athletes' body anomalies in interviews published in popular magazines such as *Die Ziet* and *Der Spiegel*, and accused her former fatherland of having a secret doping programme. The German press

---

4   Steven Ungerleider, *Faust's Gold*, St Martin's Press, 2013.

didn't take her seriously, commenting that she was just a bad loser in search of a moment of fame.

The sportswoman from Thuringia didn't give up and, after ending her competitive career, she decided, with the help of her husband, Werner Franke, to embark on a quest to collect testimonies and evidence to prove her theory of a state-sponsored doping programme in East Germany. However, during the 70s and 80s, despite some defections, it was still very difficult to find someone willing to cooperate and reveal the 'training methods' adopted by scientists and coaches and the chemical substances that circulated within the locker rooms of the GDR sports clubs. The two researchers suspected that doctors and trainers administered dangerous drugs to enhance physical performances; Franke also believed that the perpetrators probably knew about the side effects but were forced to conceal them.

Werner Franke is very well qualified to consider such assumptions as he is professor of molecular biology at Heidelberg University; he actually specialised in the study of sport-related drugs and is also director of the Cancer Research Centre. After marrying Brigitte Berendonk in 1975, he began to fight a long ideological battle against the use and abuse of pharmaceutical substances by East German athletes; he feared that in the long run they might suffer from some unwanted collateral damage. Thanks to his wife's life experience and the information gathered from a few deserters from the East, Franke began to develop a rough idea about the possible 'experiments' carried out on the athletes who lived beyond the Iron Curtain. Unfortunately, confirming theories and suppositions was nearly impossible in the secretive and secluded German Democratic Republic; Franke and Berendonk's suggestion had to remain an educated guess until 1989.

With the fall of the Berlin Wall, and the subsequent collapse of the German Democratic Republic, Brigitte

Berendonk and Werner Franke begin a frantic search among the original documents in the *Stasi* archives; their intention is to find evidence linked to the state-sponsored doping programme. It's a race against time; the two researchers know too well that many documents have been destroyed and others still in existence face the same fate. Besides, there is a realistic chance that the crimes committed will go unpunished because of the statute of limitations.

During the first stages of their investigation, Berendonk and Franke stumble across a note related to an interesting work by an elusive scientist named Hartmut Riedel: a thesis on the effects of Oral-Turinabol, an anabolic steroid, on the athletes' performances. The number of people involved in the study seems quite large: finding Dr Riedel's work would open the access to a list of athletes and possibly the method used to administer the steroids to them and eventual side effects. Unfortunately, the diligent officers of the *Ministerium* acted rapidly and managed to erase any evidence of that thesis.[5]

In parallel with their search for classified files, Franke and Berendonk also gather confidential testimonies from former athletes and personalities implicated to some degree with the GDR sports machine. Most of the information looks interesting and provides a good contribution to the understanding of certain pharmaceutical practices that took place beyond the Wall; unfortunately, none of the interviewed individuals will provide factual evidence to support their stories. Some of them, after revealing their version of the events, decide to pull back and retract their statements.[6]

In short, six months after the opening of the Brandenburg Gate, what the two investigators have in their hands is just

5   Brigitte Berendonk, *Doping. Von der Forschung zum Betrug*, Springer, 1991.
6   Ibid.

a few clues, some confessions but very little documented evidence.

In the autumn of 1990, something unexpected happens. Dr Manfred Höppner, one of the most prominent figures in the GDR sports system, and in charge of the research centre in Kreischa, near Dresden, decides to come forward and reveal everything he knows about the state-sponsored doping programme. He sells 10,000 pages of classified documents taken from the archives of the laboratory he directed to the popular magazine *Stern*. It is not known if Höppner is confessing out of guilt and to clear his conscience or for other reasons – the fact is that in issue 49 (1990) of the Hamburg-based publication we can read, for the first time, everything about the incredible doping system developed in the GDR.[7]

The article is sensational and its echo reverberates throughout the world. Everyone can now see the evidence, from a reliable source, of what Werner Franke and Brigitte Berendonk had suspected for years but were never able to prove, i.e. the continuous and structured administration of doping in East Germany since the end of the 1960s. Furthermore, from 1974 the drug programme was implemented according to rules conceived by the government itself.

It isn't a conspiracy theory anymore: it is real.

In the startling revelations included in the magazine there is also a list of athletes who are still active (at the end of 1990), who the magazine claims had been involved, knowingly or unknowingly, in the state-sponsored doping programme; among them are swimmer Kristin Otto, sprinter Heike Drechsler and shot putters Udo Beyer and Ulf Timmermann. All have denied knowingly taking drugs. Höppner's memorandum also reports in detail dates, personalised training programmes, types and amounts of drugs given to

---

7   Randy Harvey, *German Steroid Scandal Unfolds Rapidly*, Los Angeles Times, 4 December 1990.

the athletes and other relevant information.[8] These documents are what Brigitte Berendonk and Werner Franke have been looking for. The data reported gives them the information they need to search for other clues.

Margitta, the first

Manfred Höppner's documents show, beyond a reasonable doubt, the existence of a sophisticated pharmaceutical programme aimed mainly at a rapid growth of the athletes' muscular system and a fast recovery from fatigue, in order to improve sporting performance. Particularly, a team of scientists in Leipzig, led by Dr Karl-Heinz Bauersfeld, had spent years studying the effects of a male hormone like testosterone (an anabolic steroid) on the bodies of female athletes and, consequently, on their sports results; they had found out that synthetic steroids could significantly improve women's performances.[9]

Some athletes, during the 1960s, had occasionally tried by themselves to enhance their performance through the use of certain drugs (e.g. amphetamines), but the intention of the GDR officials was to 'regulate' scientifically the procedures of the intake of those substances and their elimination from the body, in order to maximise results and avoid being caught out by the doping control officers.

The first controlled experiment was carried out on a shot-putter, Margitta Gummel. The Magdeburg-born athlete was given 10mg of Oral-Turinabol (testosterone) per day, during the three months preceding the Olympic Games in Mexico City, and, incredibly, her shot-putting distance improved by about two metres.

---

8   Jutta Heess, *Sichtung und Wahrheit*, Die Zeit, 7 March 2002.
9   *Die Doping-Erkenntnisse der DDR*, Berliner Zeitung, 11 April 1994.

Testosterone is mainly a male hormone, present in variable concentration, between 270 and 1,070ng/dl (nanograms per decilitre), whilst in women its occurrence is about 7–8 times lower. When a female's level of this molecule is increased, her muscle mass and level of aggression also increase as a result, making her physically and psychologically more competitive. The strengthening due to testosterone earned Margitta a gold medal in Mexico, with a world record distance of 19.61m. The experiment was a complete success!

After 'employing' Margitta Gummel as a guinea pig, the methodical implementation of the new doping protocols was extended to other muscular disciplines, such as swimming, weightlifting and other track and field events. In the following Olympic Games, the GDR athletes attained phenomenal achievements; in just eight years the number of gold medals won increased from nine (Mexico City, 1968) to 20 (Munich, 1972) and then 40 (Montréal, 1976) – most of those medals were won by women, despite the fact that the number of events available to them was fewer than for men.

However, after Montréal '76 the element of surprise was finished. Rumours relating to the unnatural body size of the female athletes started to circulate among sports specialists; also, in the rare interviews the East German athletes gave to the press, they spoke in deep, guttural voices, which didn't sound exactly feminine. The IAAF began to increase dope testing and the East German authorities thought they should review their protocols (as we'll see in the following chapters) and suspend the programme for a little while.

Nevertheless, the data collected during the early 70s was good enough to draw a conclusion on the study and application of synthetic steroids: in terms of performance enhancement, drugs were immensely more effective on women than men. In 1977, Dr Höppner reported in detail such findings: 'At the moment, steroids are applied to all Olympic sporting events, apart from sailing and gymnastics (women) ... and all national teams. ... The positive value of anabolic steroids for the development of a top performance is undisputed. ... Performances could be improved with the support of these drugs within four years as follows: shot put (men) 2.5-4m, (women) 4.5–5m; discus throw (men) 10–12m, (women) 11–20m; hammer throw (men) 6–10m; javelin throw (women) 8–15m; 400m (women) 4–5 seconds; 800m (women) 5–10 seconds; 1,500m (women) 7–10 seconds. ... Extraordinary rates of increase in performance were also noted in women's swimming events. ... From our experiences so far, it can be concluded that women have the greatest advantage from treatments with anabolic hormones.'[10]

The incredible revelations published by *Stern* spark a chain reaction of interviews and further confessions by other GDR exponents; almost at the same time, another popular West German magazine, *Der Spiegel*, prints an interview with former swimmer Raik Hannemann, who admits to having taken steroids for years: 'We all took them. I tried many of them because I wanted privileges, such as an apartment, a place at a university and a car.'[11]

In a country where people lived almost isolated from the rest of the planet, athletes had the rare privilege of being able to travel around the world and to come into contact with the political and social systems of other nations; to them, the countries of the Western Bloc appeared particularly intriguing. Olympic silver medallist Katharina Bullin, a volleyball player, remarks on the importance of those privileges: 'We could go abroad and visit capitalist countries. When I was 15 I went to Italy! Going to Italy was impossible for the common citizen. We enjoyed a lot of bonuses, like

---

10 Manfred Höppner's report to *Stasi, Unterlagen-Archiv*, 3 March, 1977 (pp. 243–44), published (among others) in M. McClusky, *Faster, Higher, Stronger*, Penguin, 2014.

11 Randy Harvey, *World Sports Scene: German Steroid Scandal Unfolds Rapidly*, Los Angeles Times, 4 December 1990.

exotic food (oranges, bananas); sometimes I would secretly bring some home.'[12]

In November 1990 *Der Spiegel* published an interview with Michael Regner, a swimming trainer particularly known for his motivational skills who worked for the club ASK Potsdam. At the beginning of his career, Regner was moved by great ideals and couldn't wait to start training world-class swimmers like Kristin Otto, Susanne Börnike, Grit Müller and Diana Block. He was disillusioned to find all the girls had been doped without their consent: 'One day I was summoned by Dr Jochen Neubauer, managing director of the club; in the privacy of his office, he gave me an envelope containing some blue pills. Neubauer explained to me that I was supposed to give half a pill per day to each athlete. He said that their content was top secret. The plan was to grind and dissolve them in a vitamin drink – the girls would never have found out. They forced me to sign a secrecy agreement: I couldn't reveal anything about it or they would have punished me.'[13] After confessing his involvement in the doping plan, Michael Regner flees to New Zealand, to get a job as a trainer with the national swimming team.

As the first revealing confessions begin to circulate among the West German media, they are followed by more and more interesting disclosures. However, it is only fair to acknowledge that the first real admissions by East German athletes had occurred back in 1978, during very difficult times. Sprinter Renate Neufeld had in fact disclosed a great deal about the illegal doping practices taking place at her club, TSC Berlin, after defecting to West Germany with the help of her fiancé, Pentscho Spassov, a TV commentator from Bulgaria. Renate's flight had negative consequences for her family: her father,

---

12 Interview (abridged version) in the documentary *Doping for Gold*, PBS, 2007.

13 Interview (abridged version) in *Delikate Frage*, Der Spiegel, 4 February 1991.

a teacher, was fired, and her sister, a handball player, was expelled from her club.[14] Neufeld's story appeared in the newspaper *Die Welt*, in the form of an interview edited by Willi Knecht, a consummate RIAS[15] journalist. However, as Knecht had paid Neufeld for the interview, and as *Die Welt* was after all an anti-communist newspaper, readers doubted the sprinter's story and the topic soon fell into obscurity.[16]

Renate Neufeld was not the only sportsperson to flee East Germany in the late 70s; between 1976 and 1979, some 15 athletes managed to cross the East–West border. Among them, ski jumper Hans-Georg Aschenbach was one of the few who tried to reveal what was going on in East Germany: 'Those who compete in ski jumping start getting injections in their knee from the age of 14; this is because the training regime is too intense. For each Olympic champion produced, there are some 350 disabled sportsmen. I know some gymnasts who, by the 18th year of age, need to wear a bust correction belt because their spine and ligaments are totally worn out. The intense training has even made some of them mentally unstable – a consequence much worse than having a "cracked spine".'[17] Unfortunately, his words remained confined to a few lines in some newspapers.

Neufeld and Assenbach's accounts seemed more than enough to start an investigation by the IOC, the International Olympic Committee, but the time was not right to delve into a problem which might have ruined the feeble balance of political relations between states. We were living in the Cold War era, after all.

---

14 *DDR: Schluck Pillen oder kehr Fabriken aus*, Der Spiegel, 19 March 1979.

15 *Rundfunk im Amerikanischer Sektor*, a US–West German radio station which broadcast in Eastern territory as well.

16 Michael Getler, *Athlete Who Fled E. Germany Cites Forced Drug Use*, The Washington Post, 29 December 1978.

17 Interview in *Le Figaro*, 19 January 1989.

Bad Saarow

Although many important documents had been destroyed, these interviews prove to be very useful, driving Franke and Berendonk towards the right path; their plan is to collate enough evidence to prosecute the people responsible for the state-sponsored doping system in East Germany.

The mosaic tesserae starts to show an interesting pattern that conveys the proportions of the 'athlete's building programme' conceived by the East German officials and scientists. Former doctors and coaches' confessions are certainly useful, but the two investigators also need solid evidence (official documents), in order to press charges against the right people.

In 1991, a few months after the surprising interviews appear in *Stern* and *Der Spiegel*, Franke and Berendonk come across the most incredible and unexpected find of their investigation, thanks to an anonymous tip.[18] Inside one of the rooms of the military hospital in Bad Saarow, near Berlin, they discover a massive *Stasi* archive which contains thousands of documents, all faithful copies of those once stored at the Ministry for State Security, which had been destroyed.[19]

Ironically, one of the most sinister aspects of the *Stasi* – the obsession with recording and cataloguing everything to do with the East German citizens' lives in order to satisfy an almost pathological desire for bureaucratic completeness – eventually allowed the two researchers to recover about 150 classified documents relating to the doping programme. The majority of the work was carried out at the Research Institute for Physical Culture and Sports in Leipzig, and at the Central Doping Control Laboratory in Kreischa. The Bad Saarow find is of the utmost importance; the entire secret state-sponsored

18 Interview in *The Perfect Race, 20/20*, by Elizabeth Vargas, produced by Barbara Walters and Janice Tomlin, ABC TV, October 2000.
19 Mike Dennis and Jonathan Grix, *Sport Under Communism – Behind the East German Miracle*, Palgrave Macmillan, 2012.

doping programme is found in these files, including detailed information on relevant people, dates, medical reports, scientific studies, results, side effects and damages. We will see and discuss these findings in the following chapters.[20]

A few months after the Bad Saarow discovery, German Chancellor Helmut Kohl gives Franke and Berendonk the authorisation to study all the files found there. What they find goes beyond their own expectations. Other than the elusive Dr Riedel's thesis, they exhume tons of perfectly preserved and well-organised folders – an infernal collection of disturbing documentary material that will open the gates of hell.

---

20 Werner Franke, Brigitte Berendonk, *Hormonal doping and androgenization of athletes: a secret program of the German Democratic Republic government*, Clinical Chemistry 43:7 1262–1279, Doping in Sports (1997).

2.

STAATSPLANTHEMA 14.25

ONCE THEY have removed the thick layer of dust covering the folders hidden at Bad Saarow, Brigitte Berendonk and Werner Franke soon realise they have just found a cornucopia of information about the GDR state-sponsored doping programme. Hundreds of sports events, from the early 1960s onward, have been meticulously catalogued; for each of them it is possible to read the athletes' names, the particular drug they took and its dosage. In short, it is a collection of files that reveals to the world the twisted system that poisoned many innocent teenagers, viciously sacrificed on the altar of an ill-conceived state plan.

The core of these documents refers to a project launched in 1974 by high-ranking government and Socialist Party officials: its codename was *Staatsplanthema* (State Plan) *14.25,* a secret scheme which had been conceived back in 1964 by Dr Hans Schuster, one of the leading scientific executives in GDR sport. Schuster was considered an excellent, strategic-thinking planner in top-class sport; he suggested that there should be an official organisation or a body in the GDR to take on the task of combatting the use of doping. Under this guise, intensive research and development of necessary drug preparations would then be possible. Schuster thought that this project could only succeed with *Stasi* supervision, so he proposed his idea to Erich Mielke, the powerful head of the East German Ministry for State Security. Mielke initially intended to use doping to enhance the performances of his Dynamo Berlin sports club, but after a while, in the early 1970s, he decided to extend the plan to all sports federations in the GDR. Dr Hans Schuster coordinated the entire project through the Research Institute for Physical Culture and Sport (FKS) at the DHfK in Leipzig, which he headed from its founding in 1969 to 1990.[21]

The plan was implemented by unscrupulous politicians, corrupt bureaucrats, dishonest scientists and deceitful trainers, all supporting a hideous programme whose main purpose was to promote the rise of East Germany's international prestige through amazing sports results.

The German Democratic Republic was generally considered by the international community to be just a satellite state under the heavy influence of the Soviet Union. The East German leaders knew that their country was not highly regarded by the other nations and during the 60s they tried harder and harder to put their fatherland on the map. Sport was seen as an efficient propaganda means, probably the only one, to help the small European country to assert itself before the world. If until 1974 there had been some unsystematic doping procedures in place in certain sports clubs, thanks to the personal initiative of some athletes or trainers, with *Staatsplanthema 14.25* the pharmaceutical aspect of the East German sports development became regulated by law.

The Bad Saarow files provide plenty of information on the genesis of *superathletes* and on the strategies implemented to avoid failing drug tests. The key research locations were in Leipzig and Kreischa. The fact that synthetic anabolic steroids, developed in 1935 by German chemist and Nobel laureate Adolf Butenandt, could enhance muscular strength and endurance had been known since the time of the Second World War. According to anecdotal accounts, Hitler's

---

21 Giselher Spitzer, *Doping in der DDR*, Sportverlag Strauss, 2018.

scientists used to provide abundant doses to *Wehrmacht* and *SS* officers with the purpose of increasing their resistance and aggression in battle.[22] As if to follow in the steps of a wicked tradition, which had its roots in German territory, those chemicals were 'exhumed' and modified to improve the East German athletes' performances and, consequently, transform a small USSR satellite state into a world sports superpower.

The anabolic steroid in question was commercially known as Oral-Turinabol and was produced by VEB Jenapharm, a pharmaceutical company founded in 1950. Jenapharm has always said it did nothing wrong. It claimed Oral-Turinabol was legally approved in the GDR and available on the market for medical treatment, but it was misused by sports physicians and trainers. One of the most important features of the drug, other than generating muscular augmentation, was to prevent the negative effects of prolonged exercise; i.e. muscles tended to become stronger, instead of wearing out because of exhaustion. As well as being administered steroids, all athletes were subjected to a very tough training regime, which was an important component behind their victories – drugs alone would never have created so many world-class champions.[23]

A careful analysis of the *Stasi* declassified files shows vividly how the architects of *Staatsplanthema 14.25* were aware of the fact that Oral-Turinabol caused undesirable psychological side effects on the athletes' mind, such as a generic sense of omnipotence and a relatively strong sexual drive in women.[24] After a year of experiments, the doctors noticed that several

---

22   Sports Illustrated, *How we got here*, Arena Group, 11 March 2008.

23   Mike Dennis and Jonathan Grix, *Sport Under Communism – Behind the East German Miracle*, Palgrave Macmillan, 2012.

24   Werner Franke and Brigitte Berendonk, *Hormonal doping and androgenization of athletes: a secret program of the German Democratic Republic government*, Clinical Chemistry 43:7 1262–1279, Doping in Sports (1997).

boys and girls developed worrying physiological conditions: liver problems, cardiac arrhythmia, anomalous concentrations of cholesterol, irregular menstrual cycles and unusual growth of genital organs in girls (but atrophy in boys). Despite the disturbing data, no athlete was ever informed, or asked to abandon the programme. The doctors were positive that if the steroids were administered under controlled cycles, the physical and mental consequences for the athletes would be acceptable.[25]

The State Plan had established that, in order to maximise their effects, drugs had to be given in series of four-week cycles; the athletes would take 1mg doses of Oral-Turinabol (pink pill) alternating with 5mg doses (blue pill). Doses could vary, depending on the type of sport and competition. Athletes with higher hopes of reaching the final stages of important competitions were subjected to more intense cycles.

The extraordinary wins of the East Germans from 1968 to 1973 had alerted the International Olympic Committee. The highest international sports authority moved rapidly and decided in 1974 to include anabolic steroids in the list of prohibited substances; contextually, they also improved the efficacy of the doping test system by employing sophisticated technologies, such as mass spectrometers and gas chromatography instruments, in order to obtain a more accurate chemical analysis. These were devised by West German chemist, and former professional cyclist, Manfred Donike and Hewlett-Packard. The IOC increased the number of tests per year and introduced urine analysis. Ironically, one of the international laboratories chosen by the IOC to examine the urine samples was actually at Kreischa, right in the hands of East German scientists.[26] Dietrich

---

25 Mike Dennis and Jonathan Grix, *Sport Under Communism – Behind the East German Miracle*, Palgrave Macmillan, 2012.

26 David Mottram and Neil Chester, *Drugs in Sport*, Routledge, 2015.

Behrendt, who was deputy head of the doping control centre, once admitted that, 'The laboratory was not founded with the aim of combatting doping, but to enable doping. The controls served to ensure that the anabolic doping could not be discovered.'[27]

The counter-offensive had to be swift. The new set of tests, rules and controls posed a serious risk to the state-sponsored doping system: a decisive defence plan had to be deployed as soon as possible. It was essential to recalibrate the drug administration cycles in a way that any evidence of doping would disappear before the sports event. Between 1974 and 1975, the East German researchers found out that any trace of Oral-Turinabol would be eliminated from the body after a period of 25–30 days. The assumption was therefore that all athletes should stop taking drugs a month before their competition. This supposition worked effectively on the first occasion, the European Athletics Championships in Rome (September 1974). During the event, 17 athletes from various nations tested positive for anabolic steroids: not one of them was from the GDR, although they too used that drug. East Germany topped the medal table with ten golds.[28]

The mandatory order to succeed in reaching world sporting supremacy came directly from the Politburo of the Socialist Party, explicitly the most important political organ in the German Democratic Republic; the party officers reiterated to everyone involved with the plan that it was imperative to gain international prestige by winning as many medals as possible, by any means necessary and, at the same time, to avoid the embarrassment of testing positive during drug tests. As incredible and pretentious as it may seem, things would go exactly as planned, but at what cost?

27 Grit Hartmann, *Sport-Chronik der Wende*, Deutschlandfunk, 22 August 2010.

28 Giselher Spitzer, *Doping in der DDR*, Sportverlag Strauss, 2018.

One of the *Staatsplanthema* rules stated the importance of keeping the highest level of confidentiality about the origin of the chemical substances distributed to underage athletes; teenagers weren't allowed to know anything about the type of pills they were given, and any embarrassing questions would be ignored. As per the adults, trainers sometimes disclosed that they were giving them 'supporting means' (*Unterstützende Mittel*), without specifying their nature in detail. Athletes who came to know about (or suspected) the origin of those 'means' were bound to secrecy; the penalty for discussing the 'supplements' was usually the expulsion of the students from the club and the loss of privileges for them and their families. Doctors and trainers actually did everything they could to ensure that nobody ever suspected the real nature of those coloured pills; apart from dismissing any questions by particularly curious athletes, they used to remove the tablets from their original box and wrap, so that no one could read their source or chemical composition.[29] This concealing procedure occasionally failed and some athletes found out what they were really taking. To solve the problem once and for all, the pharmaceutical company was ordered to produce testosterone tablets disguised as vitamins.[30]

As Werner Franke and Brigitte Berendonk sift through the pages of the Bad Saarow documents, they also find that many officials of various sports clubs and federations were linked to the *Stasi*; some of them were actually either agents or IM, 'unofficial collaborators'. All activities, behavioural and medical, were meticulously recorded, collated and reported to high-ranking executives. These connections created a net of secrecy and isolation around the athletes; if one of them tried

---

29 Werner Franke and Brigitte Berendonk, *Hormonal doping and androgenization of athletes: a secret program of the German Democratic Republic government*, Clinical Chemistry 43:7 1262–1279, Doping in Sports (1997).

30 Giselher Spitzer, *Doping in der DDR*, Sportverlag Strauss, 2018.

to confidentially question the system or the training methods, they would be immediately caught out.

Nothing was left to chance. All the people responsible for the running of the doping plan were professionals of the highest order. Each sports club, for instance, had one or two physicians who were in charge of monitoring athletes' progress, solving all problems linked to training and, especially, supervising the administration of the blue and pink pills. Dr Lothar Kipke was one of them; he was also a powerful supervisor of the DSSV, the swimming federation, one of the most important and medal-generating sports organisations. Kipke, as many other managers, was allegedley a *Stasi* informer[31] (codename: 'Rolf'); his associate, and one of the heads of the *Staatsplanthema*, was none other than Dr Manfred Höppner, the well-respected member of the international scientific community who decided to confess his 'accomplishments' to *Stern* magazine. He was allegedly a *Stasi* informer too (codename: 'Technik').[32]

In short, all major sports institutions were run by highly qualified, skilled and competent people, whose personalities were certainly polluted by a necessary degree of cynicism and ruthlessness; all united by two objectives: creating *superathletes* and winning medals.

The first and the last

Everything went well for years, but at some point, despite its state-of-the-art technology, the efficient GDR machine unexpectedly failed. At the European Cup in Helsinki, in 1977, shot putter Ilona Slupianek tested positive for anabolic steroids. Slupianek was disqualified and banned for one year. East German managers and officials were stunned. They

---

31   http://news.bbc.co.uk/1/hi/world/europe/733155.stm
32   Michael Butcher, *Frankenstein coaches face their accusers*, The Guardian, 19 September 1999.

had precisely calculated the body absorption and elimination cycles of the steroids: the system had been working for years without a problem. What went wrong?

The new analysis techniques devised by the IAAF had evidently improved beyond expectation and they were now threatening to expose the doping plan. A quick counter-action was urgently required.

The first step, in spring 1978, was to acquire a very expensive ($187,000) Hewlett-Packard mass spectrometer, to allow doctors to monitor more precisely the concentration of steroids in athletes' urine. Secondly, the East German authorities decided to upgrade the control measures and make them more restrictive: none of the athletes would be allowed to compete if the doping substances in their urine weren't completely eliminated.[33]

Dr Manfred Höppner was in charge of the whole organisation. Essentially, before an event all athletes had to provide their urine inside specifically designed vials; these, identified by an alphanumeric code (just to exaggerate even more the levels of secrecy of the entire operation), had to be sent to the main laboratory in Kreischa, where a team of scientists, led by Dr Claus Clausnitzer, would analyse them.[34] Clausnitzer constantly communicated with Höppner about the results by telephone. All vials and documents were finally transferred to East Berlin, to the Department of Sport Medicine, where a few selected officers could associate the codes with the athletes' names. If a test result was positive, the athlete in question would be stopped from taking part in the planned event.[35]

---

33 Tim Harris, *Sport: Almost Everything You Ever Wanted to Know*, Yellow Jersey, 2008.

34 https://www.latimes.com/archives/la-xpm-1990-12-04-sp-5768-story.html

35 Documentary *Doping for Gold*, PBS, 2007.

Hundreds of urine samples had to be tested by one laboratory just a few days before competing. The technicians at the Kreischa research centre had to complete all analyses very quickly, up to a few hours before the athletes left for the event-hosting country – there was no room for mistakes or wastes of time.

The newly acquired HP mass spectrometer proved to be very useful, with a degree of accuracy and reliability close to 100 per cent; it was in fact able to detect even infinitesimal traces of doping substances in the urine samples. This new level of efficiency led the scientists to review and implement modern steroid administration procedures, and to calibrate the timing of when to stop the treatment before competitions. Ironically, a hated capitalist country had provided the East German authorities with a really functional instrument.[36]

The spectrometer soon showed its worth. A few days before the Swimming World Championships in West Berlin, in 1978, Petra Thumer and Christiane Knacke-Sommer tested positive for nandrolone. After they failed a second, last-minute test, performed literally hours before they were due to leave for West Germany, the DSSV decided to avoid any risk and prevented the two swimmers from attending the event. The official reason for their withdrawal was 'flu'.

Up to 1978, East German scientists believed that a 30-day period was long enough for the human body to get rid of all doping substances, but the case of Thumer and Knacke-Sommer showed that certain chemicals needed more time to decompose completely. Manfred Ewald, the all-powerful sports minister, decided to temporarily suspend the doping programme for a few months whilst new guidelines and drug administration cycles were studied by scientists and trainers. The consequence of the 'hold-up' materialised

---

36 Steven Ungerleider, *Faust's Gold: Inside The East German Doping Machine*, St Martin's Press, 2013.

in the form of disappointing performances by the East Germany team at the Swimming World Championships: just one gold medal! A very poor achievement if compared with the 11 gold medals won at the Montréal Olympics two years earlier.

Franke and Berendonk continued to avidly read the declassified files, discovering that other than improving the *Staatsplanthema* protocols thanks to the HP spectrometer, the East German scientists were always working hard to study and test new drugs on the athletes; one of those substances was testosterone ester. Its main attribute was to be an undetectable alternative to the usual anabolic androgenic steroid; it could be injected into athletes of both sexes as a substitute for detectable steroids from three to four weeks before a competition until the last week before it. After 1974, it became common practice to inject testosterone ester in this way; with this substance, virilising effects on female athletes were more pronounced.[37]

At some point, a substance called mestanolone was delivered from the ZENET[38] laboratory in Jena to the Research Institute for Physical Culture and Sports (FKS) in Leipzig. This was a kind of steroid discovered in 1935 but never tested on human beings. After an initial trial on volleyball and handball players, Manfred Höppner, in a rare moment of moral decency, warned against that substance as its effects were still unknown and potentially dangerous for pregnant girls. Unfortunately, despite Höppner's warning, the drug was occasionally used by some athletes with dire consequences for their liver. Two of those athletes, hammer

---

37 Werner Franke and Brigitte Berendonk, *Hormonal doping and androgenization of athletes: a secret program of the German Democratic Republic government*, Clinical Chemistry 43:7 1262–1279, Doping in Sports (1997).

38 Central Institute for Microbiology and Experimental Therapy (*Zentralinstitut für Mikrobiologie und Experimentelle Therapie*).

throwers Detlef Gerstenberg and Uwe Beyer, died of hepatic cirrhosis, both in 1993.[39]

Another 'useful' substance that came straight from Jenapharm was epitestosterone. This was not particularly effective in enhancing sports performances but it was mainly employed as a masking agent to hide high levels of testosterone. It had been established by the IOC that the testosterone/epitestosterone ratio had to be no more than 6:1 in order to not fail a doping test; the addition of synthetic epitestosterone in the human body would obviously reduce an athlete's ratio.[40]

In the perfect world of the GDR doping system there was, however, also room for improvisation. From the Bad Saarow documents we see that, in case of emergency (i.e. urine potentially still contaminated with the presence of doping), the East German managers were instructed to use their own physiological excretion and operate a sample substitution on the go, before the analysis took place.[41]

With all these new precautions, both technological and creative, by the end of the 1970s the GDR state-sponsored doping system effectively became bulletproof. The case of Ilona Slupianek remained the first and last positive test in the whole history of the country.

The many documents retrieved by Werner Franke and Brigitte Berendonk prove beyond a shadow of a doubt that their suspicions are well-founded: a state-sponsored doping system in East Germany really existed and it was responsible

39 Frank Bachner, *Schnell die der Tod*, Der Tagesspiel, 22 September 1998.

40 Werner Franke and Brigitte Berendonk, *Hormonal doping and androgenization of athletes: a secret program of the German Democratic Republic government*, Clinical Chemistry 43:7 1262–1279, Doping in Sports (1997).

41 Steven Ungerleider, *Faust's Gold: Inside The East German Doping Machine*, St Martin's Press, 2013.

for the creation of a generation of phenomenal athletes that mesmerised and dominated the world of sports for two decades. The cheating element due to the 'pharmaceutical help' was obviously great, and so was the risk of harming young athletes, as we will see in the second part of this book.

All the material found at Bad Saarow was methodically studied, collated and promptly published in 1991 (complete with full names, dates and circumstances) by Brigitte Berendonk in her book, *Doping. Von der Forschung zum Betrug* (Doping. From Research to Fraud). Her work caused quite a stir in public opinion, and would be one of the main 'tools' that, a few years later, persuaded the authorities of unified Germany to put the East German perpetrators on trial.

3.

THE FACTORY OF CHAMPIONS

THROUGH ABOUT 150 years of professional and amateur sport, doping has always played a part. For many years, the act of enhancing a physical performance through the use of chemical substances was considered 'normal', accepted by everyone, and not perceived as a scandal. Scientific literature reports how, in the 19th century, cyclists used various stimulants, such as caffeine, morphine and alcohol. With regard to the latter, it looks like the root of the word 'doping' comes from a Dutch ethylic drink, derived from a type of South African grape's skin, called *dop*.[42]

At the Olympic Games in St Louis, in 1904, Thomas Hicks won the marathon with the support of some injections of strychnine (a poisonous substance that in small doses acts as a stimulant), administered during the race (in plain sight!), by Charles Lucas, his doctor. Lucas later wrote a scientific article concluding that, 'The marathon race, from a medical stand-point, demonstrated that drugs are of much benefit to athletes along the road, and that warm sponging is much better than cold sponging for an athlete in action.'[43] No one in the sporting or scientific community raised an eyebrow over that article. In the 1920s, however, synthetic amphetamines started to

---

42 David Mottram and Neil Chester, *Drugs in Sport*, Routledge, 2015.

43 Reported in Mark Johnson, *Spitting in the Soup: Inside the Dirty Game of Doping in Sports*, 2006.

circulate among athletes, and the IAAF, in 1928, getting worried about possible abuses by sportsmen, decided to ban them, although there weren't methods to detect the intake of the drug: respect for the rules depended entirely on an athlete's honesty. It was, therefore, a matter of ethics. Regarding ethics, in 1941, the US physiologist Dr Peter Karpovich stated that, 'The use of a substance or device which improves the physical performance of a man without being injurious to his health, can hardly be called unethical.'[44]

In those years, sportsmen were considered entertainers and, as such, it was only fair that they could express themselves (i.e. compete) to the best of their abilities, even through the use of drugs. However, in 1946 everything changed, as the newly reformed International Olympic Committee decided that anyone who used or distributed performance-enhancing drugs could not take part in the Olympic Games. Obviously, there was no objective way (for at least the next two decades) for the event organisers to check if an athlete had taken doping substances, but an important principle was established.

The dawn of cheating

Apparently, the use of anabolic steroids 'officially' started in 1954, at the World Weightlifting Championships in Vienna. During that event, the US team's doctor, John Ziegler, suspected that the Soviet Union athletes had performed exceptionally well and won several medals thanks to the aid of testosterone-based substances; he experimented a lot with anabolic steroids, but his weightlifters didn't benefit much from them. In 1958, Ziegler tried a new synthetic steroid produced by Ciba Pharmaceuticals called methandrostenolone

---

44 Mark Johnson, *Doping has always been part of the Olympics. Of course Russia got off the hook*, The Washington Post, 29 July 2016.

(marketed as Dianabol).[45] He successfully tested the effects of this new drug on himself, before administering it to the athletes. Ziegler's intentions were, however, to play safe and he insisted that the intake of the pills wouldn't harm the athletes. Unfortunately, once they discovered the 'magic' behind the pills, the US weightlifters took them indiscriminately and unsafely. In the end Ziegler became a profound critic of the same practice he started himself, but the damage was done. The substances went undetected for years, as a reliable doping test able to identify anabolic steroids wasn't ready before the Montréal Olympics, in 1976.[46]

All 'wonders of chemistry' used and abused were considered merely an expedient to cheat and win medals; nobody had ever expressed (publicly, at least) the possibility that they could damage an athlete's health. In 1960 everything changed. During the Olympic Games in Rome, Knud Enemark Jensen, a Danish cyclist, felt sick during the team time trial event. He managed to finish the race, helped by his team-mates, but died soon after. The post-mortem toxicology test revealed the presence of amphetamines (although, in recent times the reliability of that test has been criticised).[47] The doctors disagreed: some of them believed in a correlation between the presence of amphetamines and Jensen's death, whilst others denied it. Nevertheless, a debate on the danger of doping had begun in the scientific community. A few years later, the tragic death of English cyclist Tom Simpson (who had taken amphetamines) during a tough stage of the Tour de France, in 1967, pushed the sport's authorities to create a reliable doping test able to find forbidden substances in the athletes' urine.

---

45 Justin Peters, *The Man Behind the Juice*, Slate.com, 18 February, 2005.

46 David Mottram and Neil Chester, *Drugs in Sport*, Routledge, 2015.

47 D. Rosen, *Dope: A History of Performance Enhancement in Sport*, ABC Clio, 2008.

The scheme was implemented for the first time at the Giro d'Italia, in May 1968, and a few months later was widely used during the Olympic Games in Mexico City.[48]

The wonder machine

In those years, the East German authorities took advantage of the fact that doping tests were virtually non-existent, to organise a complex sporting system that merged advanced training techniques with the devious use of undetectable drugs.

The documents found by Werner Franke and Brigitte Berendonk include plenty of details of the athletes' daily routines and training programmes, as well as aspects of their private lives. One of the most important (and successful) institutions was the famous SC Dynamo Berlin; this was managed by alleged *Stasi* informants Dr Dieter Binus and trainer Rolf Gläser. After 1990, it would emerge that nearly all the club's employees had alleged connections, to various extents, with the secret police. Dr Binus took care mainly of the athletes' health conditions and was responsible for the recruitment of specialists who would deal with serious injuries; a gynaecologist was always present to assist sportswomen. Gläser's duty was to monitor the intake of drugs according to East German scientists' guidelines.[49]

The swimming department was one of the most active. Girls were recruited at the age of 11, after a very strict selection process that took into account their innate talent and body size. Once accepted, they were subjected to back-breaking training regimes developed by the club's physicians and scientists. In addition, from that moment on, their private lives came under the programme's control. Each of the girls had a personalised training plan; their results and scores were

---

48 William Fotheringham, *Put Me Back on My Bike: In Search of Tom Simpson*, Vintage Digital, 2012.

49 Steven Ungerleider, *Faust's Gold: Inside The East German Doping Machine*, St Martin's Press, 2013.

continuously analysed, in order to verify improvements or deficiencies in their performance. It was very important to understand the athletes' limits as soon as possible, in order to select suitable candidates for international competitions.

A typical day in the life of a swimmer consisted of the following programme: in the morning, swimming (8km), followed by school studies and then training in the gym before lunch; in the afternoon, a theory session and then back into the swimming pool (8km). This regime was implemented during the week, Monday to Friday, whilst on Saturday there were just the two sessions in the swimming pool. Sunday was dedicated to rest. The girls whose parents lived in the Berlin area could go and sleep at home, while those who lived further away had to live and sleep at the Seelenbinder dormitory. The strict regime that permeated the athletes' lives is summarised well by volleyball player Katharina Bullin: 'School. Training. School. Training … They always gave us orders to follow. "Put that hat on or you'll get punished … Wear that shirt or you'll get punished … After the 1st of October, don't eat ice cream or you'll get punished …" We worked hard all the time and we never had free time.'[50]

Occasionally, the athletes suspended their usual school term to attend intensive training programmes that would occur in remote places, such as Lindow and Kienbaum. Four times a year, they had to go and train at high altitude locations, such as Rabenberg and Belmeken (in Bulgaria), to improve the oxygenation of their muscles. In the 1980s, some East German teams would go and train in Mexico.

Physicians and trainers had always agreed that intense muscular efforts had to be followed by a rest period to recover from tiredness. The incredible 'resources' developed by the German Democratic Republic had succeeded in overturning that simple sporting principle by eliminating the need to

---

50 Interview in the documentary *Doping for Gold*, PBS, 2007.

rest. First of all, among the supplements prepared for the athletes there was a natural cocktail called Dynvital, a mixture of various vitamins C, B, E and B6, and other substances including iron, magnesium and egg albumen. Nothing illegal, so far, but they were just the starter on a more complex 'menu' containing a list of indefinite (to the athletes, at least) pharmaceutical compounds. Apart from the chemical support, there were also sessions of electrical muscle stimulation, followed by injections of glucose and alpha-lipoic acid.

Nothing was left to chance, not even control of the sportswomen's menstrual cycle. In fact, there was dedicated monitoring of the girls' hormonal processes; scientists tried to understand if there could be any negative interference by the cycle on the athletes' performances and their mood. It was essential to know their menstruation dates, to minimise its effect on the races' outcomes. To that end, German doctors distributed contraceptive pills, to enable them to predict and regularise the girls' periods and therefore reduce their negative effects on competitions.

Manfred Ewald, an influential member of the Socialist Unity Party and president of the DTSB (German Gymnastics and Sports Federation), had the task of guaranteeing the implementation of the *Staatsplanthema*'s directives. The DTSB supervised all sport associations through men connected to the SKS (State Committee for Physical Culture and Sport) and the SMD (Sports Medical Service of the GDR). One of the key centres of the sport system was the Central Institute for Sport Medicine (ZI), whose headquarters were in Kreischa: this was a very advanced doping control laboratory, officially recognised by the International Olympic Committee during the 1970s. Here, as we have seen before, under the direction of Dr Claus Clausnitzer (a *Stasi* agent, codename: 'Meschke'), drugs which could prove useful to enhance the athletes' performances were analysed and tested. Another important laboratory was the

Central Institute for Microbiology and Experimental Therapy (ZIMET) in Jena, directed by Hans Knöll.

In terms of technical preparation, the most significant institute was perhaps the *Deutsche Hochschule für Körperkultur* (DHfK), in Leipzig, the place where trainers were forged, after a tough four-year university-level course. At the DHfK, coaches-to-be would study recruitment techniques, training methods and drug administration schemes for children. The facilities were the most technologically advanced in the world. Among the modern structures there was even a 'swimming channel', a sort of elongated bathtub in which water flowed in the opposite direction to that of the athlete, who would swim against the current. The tub was equipped with cameras which would record in slow motion the swimmer's movements, in order to analyse their posture and limb movements and correct any errors. The channel was often used to simulate races; in such cases, the speed of the current would gradually increase towards the end to help the swimmer to develop the habit of making an extra effort in the final metres. Former GDR swimmer Ute Krause highlights the harshness of the training: 'We had to swim and swim … until the ring of the bell. At some point we would run out of oxygen, our lungs were about to blow up and muscles ached. At the end of the day, we were all very tired.'[51]

Obviously, the intensive training methods represented only one side of the athletes' building programme; the other side of the coin was, as already mentioned, the pharmaceutical part, essentially based on the production and distribution of (mainly) anabolic steroids, such as Oral-Turinabol. This darker side was in the hands of Jenapharm, the German pharmaceutical giant which provided all types of drugs to the DTSB. Dr Rainer Hartwich, a senior officer of the Socialist Party, and *Stasi* agent, was the head of the research department: 'The secrecy

---

51   Interview in the documentary *Doping for Gold*, PBS, 2007.

of our studies was of vital importance; if anything had leaked, other countries could have taken advantage of our discoveries and made their athletes as competitive as ours.'[52] To that end, in official documents all doping substances were referred to as UM (*Unterstützende Mittel*, i.e. 'supportive means'). They were mainly steroids such as nandrolone esters, testosterone, amphetamines and oxytocins.[53]

Among the doctors, scientists, officers and trainers, there were more than 3,000 *Stasi* agents; the athletes had to be careful about their private conversations as they could be secretly overheard. Any person who said anything against the system would be punished and expelled from the club. The high level of confidentiality made it possible for the doping programme to remain secret for many years. Even when Jenapharm, at some point, produced the STS 6-4-6 mestanolone, a new steroid which caused serious virilising effects, that information was made available only to a restricted group of officers. On that occasion, because of a lack of experimental data, Dr Hartwich recommended not using the drug, but Manfred Ewald, the sports minister, ordered 63,000 doses![54]

In the mid-80s, the GDR authorities realised that anabolic steroids alone might have become obsolete or not good enough for enhancing the athletes' performances, either because other countries had found an efficient way to use them and/or because the doping test system had improved. It was therefore imperative to create new, more efficient and undetectable drugs. The new doping frontier took athletes towards

---

52 Ibid, and www.espn.co.uk/olympics/news/story?id=2048448

53 Werner Franke and Brigitte Berendonk, *Hormonal doping and androgenization of athletes: a secret program of the German Democratic Republic government*, Clinical Chemistry 43:7 1262–1279, Doping in Sports (1997).

54 Steven Ungerleider, *Faust's Gold: Inside The East German Doping Machine*, St Martin's Press, 2013.

innovative substances such as growth hormones (somatotropin and erythropoietin) or ground-breaking techniques such as the haemotransfusion. Somatotropin looked like the right drug to be used (alone or in combination with steroids) and was injected into the bodies of unaware athletes, in order to increase their muscle mass. Manfred Höppner, the top GDR sports doctor, had read about somatotropin's potential in a Western scientific magazine and had decided straight away to order the Kreischa laboratory to synthesise it.[55] The danger posed by this substance was that, if taken in excess, it could cause permanent body deformities; besides, there were issues with its safety since it was extracted from cadavers![56]

Towards the end of the 80s, growth hormones were mainly injected into the knees of athletes involved in winter sports and into the joints of female gymnasts, usually to make them recover faster from injuries. The so-called 'blood doping', employed to increase the oxygen concentration in muscles, was never really used in the GDR, as doctors refused to perform such a technique. Besides, more and more athletes started to be wary of the many 'supportive means' that circulated at the sports clubs; a blood transfusion process would have been too obvious and complex to make the athletes believe that they were just taking vitamins. The fall of the Berlin Wall, in 1989, mercifully put an end to the spasmodic quest for the perfect chemical formula ... in East Germany, at least.

Regarding doping-induced health consequences, what emerged (see next chapter) has more to do with a disturbing phenomenon of human engineering rather than sport itself: disproportionate muscle growth, hirsutism, depression, permanent damage to vital organs (mainly heart and liver) and virilisation of female bodies. 'One of the main long-standing

---

55   Pamphlet *Staatsdoping in der DDR*, Die Landesbeauftragte für Mecklenburg-Vorpommern für die Unterlagen des Staatssicherheitsdienstes der ehemaligen DDR 2017.

56   Ibid.

negative consequences of muscle growth,' highlights Brigitte Berendonk, 'is the fact that tendons can't grow at the same pace, i.e. with the same strength and flexibility. Many athletes who took anabolic steroids during their career have in fact sustained tendon injuries. A few years after the end of their career, many have developed joint-related problems, especially in their knees.'[57] Werner Franke adds that virilisation, due to the constant and progressive intake of anabolic steroids, is irreversible; other than the annoying problem of extra hair, the muscle structure of the female body would grow and remain that of a man, even after stopping taking drugs. Years after the collapse of East Germany, some sportswomen would compete for the united Germany, taking advantage of a superior muscle mass compared to that of other countries' athletes.[58]

Naturally, not all athletes who took (forcibly or not) doping substances were able to excel in their own sport specialism. For every three athletes who qualified for an international competition, there were tens who didn't even manage to participate at national level: the inner rivalry within a sports club and between sports clubs was fierce. Many coaches tried everything they could to gain glory and success and they often pushed their health supervisor to obtain more 'magic pills' to give to their athletes. After all, only top results (i.e. medals) would bring bonuses such as a salary increase and other privileges of a social nature. This competitive climate caused, in some cases, an indiscriminate rise in the distribution of drugs to the athletes; those extra chemical substances often came from the black market and this worried the GDR authorities enormously. Even Manfred Höppner expressed, at some point, his concern in a report he sent to the *Stasi*: 'Testosterone is being injected in irresponsible amounts, even

---

57   Werner W. Franke, Brigitte Berendonk, *Hormonal doping and androgenization of athletes: a secret program of the German Democratic Republic government*, Clinical Chemistry, Vol. 43, N.7, July 1997.
58   Ibid.

before competitions in which it is not so important to achieve record-breaking performances.'[59]

During important sport events, Höppner, who was also a member of the doping control committee, did his best to protect his athletes by swapping their urine with a 'clean' sample, if necessary. The 'factory of champions', other than creating *superathletes*, made sure it preserved its aura of invincibility and honesty through investments in research and a certain level of corruption, the extent of which has never been clear. In fact, doping tests, thanks to East German scientists' and officers' tentacular dirty hands, had become virtually ineffective.

The human guinea pigs

We now know that each athlete had a secret personalised plan where every gram of doping was carefully weighed against a physical training programme. Depending on the athlete's sports discipline, sex, age, height, weight and other parameters, a list of drugs (and their relative amounts) was scientifically devised and promptly provided. The question researchers have been trying to answer for a while is: how did doctors know the exact type and the quantity of doping to give to a certain athlete? The answer to this query has emerged only recently, and it is really disturbing as it has very little to do with moral scientific research and a lot to do with a rare and rather cruel case of human experimentation.

Exposing valued GDR athletes to trial-and-error tests was out of the question; the East German authorities couldn't afford to waste precious 'raw material' (i.e. promising young talents) just to verify if a certain chemical compound would work or not. To prevent the athletes from getting the wrong amount of a drug, and putting their career at risk, others had to serve in order to guarantee the success of swimmers and

---

59   Ibid.

sprinters. The Ministry of Sport decided therefore to launch a secret parallel programme where amateur athletes were used instead; scientists were free to carry out every test available on them. The programme was extremely well concealed, to the point that the laboratories were located in the basement of the Sports Institute building, away from other employees, with windowless walls and permanent (and rather depressing) neon lighting. Experiments and procedures, which took place at the DHfK in Leipzig under the supervision of Dr Hermann Buhl, were even recorded on film in 1976; this was intended for information for the state leadership only. Ruth Wolker, a journalist who shot the movie under conditions of maximum security, said: 'Everything had to be done discreetly; I was not allowed to talk about it, if I valued my career. The film was ordered by the DTSB as propaganda means to convince the SED Politburo to invest more and more money into sports.'[60]

The film has recently been found and broadcast as part of a documentary ('*Geheimsache Doping: Menschenversuche – Die heimlichen Experimente im DDR-Sport*') by the German TV Channel ARD.[61] One of the athletes that appears in the original film is Hans-Albrecht Kühne, a student journalist and an amateur long-distance runner back in the 1970s. Kühne, tracked down by the ARD investigative journalists, tells the press about his horrible experience. He was essentially convinced to become an 'experimental subject' for patriotic reasons; in exchange he would get state-of-the-art medical assistance, excellent food and, of course, a small amount of money. Kühne becomes quite emotional when he recalls his involvement in the programme: 'Nobody knew that there were people like me who were "test pilots"; it's important that people talk about it. ... It is part of the overall picture of

---

60 *Menschenversuche im DDR-Sport: Fragen und Antworten zur Recherche*, Sportschau, 26 February 2021.
61 Hajo Seppelt, Josef Opfermann and Jörg Mebus, *Menschenversuche für Medaillen*, Tagesschau, 26 February 2021.

competitive sport in the GDR. My body's reactions to training were carefully recorded; they were extremely useful as the relative analysis and conclusions drawn by the doctors could be used and applied to competitive athletes.'[62] Kühne took part in the secret programme for three years.

Other than testing Kühne over various distances, Dr Buhl and his team would frequently perform biopsies, collecting muscle and liver tissues. This procedure was extremely painful as it was carried out with the athlete wide awake – this method is actually shown in the film and it is hard to watch. The biopsies were needed to analyse the effect of the different drugs that were (secretly) given to Kühne; the athlete was unaware of the fact that he was being used to test different types of doping. Among those substances, he got injections of psychotropic drugs, the anabolic steroid Depot-Turinabol and the highly dangerous (and not approved for use on humans) STS 6-4-8.[63] With time, the athlete would develop severe kidney pain, swelling of the testicles and depression. The biopsies also destroyed the lymphatic system in his left leg.

Albrecht Kühne was not the only one to be used as a test subject: the experimental group included runner Bernd Moormann, who recalls being invited by some sport doctors to take part in the programme: 'I thought it was a good idea, but in the end I was the one to feel the pain while it was the top athletes who boarded the planes.' Another 'human guinea pig' was swimmer Jens Beckert; he was 17 at the time but he remembers distinctly that in his group there were 11 to 13-year-old children and they were subjected to biopsies as well. Beckert at some point understood what was happening and started to spit out the pills. After an international event, he tried to defect to Czechoslovakia but he was caught by the

---

62   Hajo Seppelt, Josef Opfermann and Jörg Mebus, *Menschenversuche für Medaillen*, Tagesschau, 26 February 2021.

63   *Steroidtestsubstanz* (Steroid Test Substance).

police and sentenced to one and a half years in jail, before being ransomed by West Germany.[64]

The *Stasi* archives confirm that this clandestine programme was extended to different categories of non-competitive athletes: 'students', 'amateur athletes', 'athletes in non-performance training', 'performance-oriented athletes' and even army soldiers. The aim of these tests was, obviously, to enhance top athletes' performances. In the interview, Albrecht Kühne reports how Dr Buhl praised him and remarked on the fact that his dedication, being a long-distance runner, would have been of great benefit to Waldemar Cierpinski, the famous runner who won the Olympic marathon in 1976 and 1980.

The person responsible for executing the programme, Dr Hermann Buhl, died in 2014 but his assistant, Jochen Scheibe, is still alive. After the reunification of the two Germanys, he has enjoyed a quite successful career as a highly respected sports doctor and a consultant for the Mecklenburg-Vorpommern parliament as a doping expert. Interviewed by the ARD journalists, he has denied any involvement with the state-sponsored doping programme.

The most incredible aspect of this story is that amateur athletes haven't been entitled to any compensation, as that is reserved for competitive athletes.[65] It is not clear how many people were used in this cruel programme, but Anne Drescher, state commissioner for Mecklenburg-Vorpommern for the GDR Offences, has speculated that several hundred amateur athletes were probably recruited into the programme;[66] and most of them might not even know that one of the possible

---

64 *Menschenversuche im DDR-Sport: Fragen und Antworten zur Recherche*, Sportschau, 26 February 2021.

65 We'll discuss the organisation Doping-Opfer-Hilfe in the final chapter.

66 *Menschenversuche im DDR-Sport: Fragen und Antworten zur Recherche*, Sportschau, 26 February 2021.

reasons for their poor health is a secret plan that started 50 years ago. Fortunately, in March 2021, in light of the ARD documentary, Doping-Opfer-Hilfe – the organisation that provides support to state-sponsored doping victims – started to discuss with the German government the possibility of extending compensation payments to amateur athletes.[67]

If it is bad enough becoming a national hero with permanent health problems, it has to be mockingly dreadful being constantly in pain and having lived a life in total obscurity. It would be refreshing to see that a piece of investigative journalism might prove to be pivotal in acknowledging those amateur athletes' sacrifice and making their lives better.

---

67 Pressemitteilung des Doping-Opfer-Hilfe e.V. vom 15. März 2021. Doping-Opfer-Hilfe e.V. fordert Entfristung aller Entschädigungsleistungen für Opfer des DDR-Staatsdopings. Press release D-O-H website, March 2021.

4.

DOPINGPROZESS: ACT I

BETWEEN 1989 and 1997, Werner Franke and Brigitte Berendonk succeed in collecting, cataloguing and publishing hundreds of documents related to the state-sponsored doping programme devised and implemented by the German Democratic Republic. Above all, they bring together important testimonies from many athletes who were involved in various competitions in the previous 30 years. The significant quantity of documents and the large number of key witnesses is deemed enough to take most of the people responsible for the *Staatsplanthema 14.25* and its implementation to court . On 19 February 1997, hundreds of German and foreign journalists are ready to jot down in their notebooks the proceedings of the *Dopingprozess*, a trial that lasts three and a half years, hearing evidence from doctors, managers, trainers and officers who were implicated in one of the most appalling sports scandals of all time.

Michael Lehner is a well-known lawyer for clients who can afford to pay very high fees but, in this instance, having been moved by the athletes' personal stories, he decides to offer his services for free.[68]

The trial itself, just like an Olympic event, is a race against time. The judges have to take into account the legal mechanism

---

68   Steven Ungerleider, *Faust's Gold: Inside The East German Doping Machine*, St Martin's Press, 2013.

of the statute of limitations which defines the maximum time after an event within which proceedings may start. The final rulings have to be decided by 31 October 2000. According to German law, most trials have to start within five years of the offence taking place and must end within ten years. Under this rule, the *Dopingprozess* could never have begun. Fortunately, in 1993, the German parliament decided to pass a specific law (exclusively dedicated to crimes committed in the former East Germany) that extended the statute of limitations for certain offences (e.g. violations of human rights). This made it possible to prosecute the former GDR authorities.

The people (many of them are women) who decide to bear witness come from all sports but most are from swimming and athletics; their aim is not to ask for exemplary punishments for their former doctors and coaches, but to allow the truth to come out. To them, it is absolutely necessary to reveal exactly what was going on behind the closed doors of the East German sports clubs.

The trial, for the sportswomen, doesn't start well: the court orders, upon request of some of the defence lawyers, that they all undergo a gynaecological examination, to ascertain if there has been any damage to their genital organs caused by doping – the cause-effect relationship between drugs and illness is one of the aspects the trial is attempting to establish. The results are read aloud in the hall, without sparing any detail. The defence lawyers' plan is obviously to humiliate and intimidate the accusers, but these women don't intend to withdraw from the trial and are fully willing to stand up for themselves.[69]

Many of the former swimmers have been convinced to testify by Brigitte Berendonk (defended by Lehner, as well), after the publishing of her book in 1991, the previously

---

69 Steven Ungerleider, *Faust's Gold: Inside The East German Doping Machine*, St Martin's Press, 2013.

mentioned *Doping. Von der Forschung zum Betrug*. As explained, the volume contains many declassified documents found in the *Stasi* archives at Bad Saarow, and gives accounts of illegal activities perpetrated by the East German sports doctors at the expense of many athletes. The overwhelming evidence in those documents, corroborated by doping plans found in the archives of the DTSB head office, convinced many athletes to come forward and contact the book's author; their intention was to organise a class action against the key members of the East German sports structure.[70] However, the simple prospect of standing up in a court and telling their story proves to be, for many athletes, more demanding than getting ready for a 100m Olympic final; with time, some of them will choose to abandon the trial. The few who decide to remain are, however, belligerent enough to face their former doctors and coaches.

More than 100 people, between defendants and victims, are interrogated by various judges in eight different trials. Here, we are going to report the most significant testimonies.

Lothar Kipke

Among the first defendants to approach the dock is Dr Lothar Kipke, a senior physician who had a key role in the state-sponsored doping system. During the hearing, while Kipke tries to explain and justify the reasons for his actions, his statement is interrupted by a particularly irate shout: 'You knew all along! You were totally aware of the effects [of the drugs] on our body!'[71] Judge Peter Faust has to work hard to restore order in the courtroom. The shout came from Martina

---

70   '*Staatsplanthema 14.25*' *von 1988 legte exakte Anabolika-Dosen fest Doping in der DDR (4): Mißbrauch von Aufputschmittel an 13 jährige Mädchen: Kinder – Spielbälle für Mediziner und Trainer*, Berliner Zeitung, 8 April 1994.

71   (abridged version) Steven Ungerleider, *Faust's Gold: Inside The East German Doping Machine*, St Martin's Press, 2013.

Gottschalt, a former swimming champion from Magdeburg who, together with colleagues like Karen König, Kornelia Ender and Petra Schneider, has taken Lothar Kipke to court, with the assistance of Michael Lehner.

Kipke – prosaically nicknamed 'Dr Mabuse' by *Der Spiegel*'s reporters[72] – is formally accused of being responsible for the implementation of the *Staatsplanthema* and the distribution of different types of drugs to GDR athletes, between 1973 and 1989. During his career, he had been an esteemed board member of FINA, the international swimming federation, well known to his colleagues for his stance against … doping! His defence strategy is not very tough: he actually admits all 58 accusations. Kipke did approve and distribute doping substances to unaware athletes, but he takes care to specify that he didn't know about the long-term effects of those drugs on the athletes' health. Furthermore, as often happens to people in pyramidal organisations, Kipke states he was a mere executor of orders coming from powerful people above him.

Judge Faust has probably already made up his mind about Kipke when another shout from Gottschalt interrupts his train of thought: 'Look my 15-year-old son in his eyes and tell him you were just following orders!'[73] Martina Gottschalt's son, Daniel, was born with a congenital malformation in his lower limbs called clubfoot, a condition in which a newborn's feet appear to be rotated at the ankle, and point down and inwards.[74] Science hasn't been able to explain the causes of this condition, which appears in 0.1 per cent of babies, but the fact is that many former sportswomen have delivered children bearing the same deformity. Very often, their pregnancy was

---

72 Carolin Emcke and Udo Ludwig, *Blaue Bohnen von Dr. Mabuse*, Der Spiegel, 28 February 2000.

73 (abridged version) Steven Ungerleider, *Faust's Gold: Inside The East German Doping Machine*, St Martin's Press, 2013.

74 Carolin Emcke and Udo Ludwig, *Blaue Bohnen von Dr Mabuse*, Der Spiegel, 28 February 2000.

characterised by serious health problems. It is possible that because the uteruses of women who have taken anabolic steroids become smaller, the space available for the growing foetus is reduced.

At the hearing, Barbara Krause (Gottschalt's team-mate) explains she has two children, both born with clubfoot; Jutta Gottschalk (another swimmer from Magdeburg) reveals she had a lot of problems during her pregnancy and her daughter was born blind. Other former swimmers add they had to have an abortion because of a severely malformed foetus. There is probably a long list of former GDR athletes with similar problems; I highlight 'probably' because many of them preferred not to testify and, consequently, it is difficult to know the real extent of the sportswomen's health issues. Among them, for instance, we certainly know that former shot putter Margitta Pufe, whose daughter, Jacqueline, was born with a permanent paralysis on the right side of her body, refused to appear in the courtroom because she does not wish to recall her past and just wants to be left alone. We know her story through sprinter Michael Dröse, her former husband, present at the trial.[75] A lot of former athletes (and their children) are in need of medical care. What they expect from the trial is legal recognition of the physical damage they suffered because of the state-sponsored doping system, so that they may be able to get compensation that would help to pay their expensive hospital bills.[76]

As mentioned above, Kipke's defence strategy is based on his (self-proclaimed) total unawareness of the steroids' negative consequences on the athletes' bodies. Unfortunately for him, in the report-confession 'offered' by his superior, Manfred Höppner, to *Der Spiegel*, it was evident that the

---

75 Ibid.

76 Matthias Krause, *An nur einem Verhandlungstag wird DDR Schwimmver-bandsarzt Lothar Kipke zu 15 Monaten auf Bewährung verurteilt*, Berliner Zeitung, 13 January 2000.

East German sports authorities were actually aware of the harmful effects on the athletes and their offspring: 'Since the use of anabolic hormones during the first stages of pregnancy may cause malformation, we recommend the administration of birth control pills. In case of pregnancy, we suggest the medical abortion.'[77]

After two years of hearings, Judge Faust fines 'Dr Mabuse' 7,800 marks and gives him a suspended 15-month prison sentence for causing intentional harm to underage athletes through the administration of anabolic steroids. Victims' lawyer Michael Lehner, who addressed Kipke as the 'Mengele of the GDR doping system', had requested a prison term of 30 months; he deems the sentence 'embarrassing', as Kipke won't even go to jail.[78]

Martina Gottschalt is particularly angry about that decision.. Her view was that Kipke didn't show any particular remorse for what he did and pretended not to know anything about the drugs' side effects. Kipke's lawyer apologises on behalf of his client to her son, after the defendant refuses to do so. Gottschalt, bitterly, tries to explain that Judge Faust's sentence is too lenient as he appeared reluctant to dig too far in the past: 'It's all very shady. Many athletes have died from the injections. We may have many skeletons in the closet.'[79] As we'll see, that remark is not very far from the truth.

Dieter Binus and Rolf Gläser

The Binus–Gläser duo, respectively physician and coach at SC Dynamo Berlin, worked together so closely that Judge Bräutigam decides to put them in the dock together. The files

---

77 Carolin Emcke and Udo Ludwig, *Blaue Bohnen von Dr. Mabuse*, Der Spiegel, 28 February, 2000.

78 *Ex-Schwimmtrainer Kipke zu bisher höchster Strafe verurteilt*, Der Spiegel, 12 January 2000.

79 Steven Ungerleider, *Faust's Gold: Inside The East German Doping Machine*, St Martin's Press, 2013.

found in the *Stasi* archives are very clear: they show enough evidence against the two officers that a sentence for violation of human rights seems practically unavoidable. From 1975 to 1989, Dieter Binus and Rolf Gläser were responsible for the distribution and administration of doping to hundreds of underage athletes. Like Kipke, they try to defend themselves by stating that they were unaware of the drugs' side effects, but this approach is firmly dismissed by Bräutigam. The judge wants to understand why Dr Binus abused his position by 'fattening' adolescent athletes with synthetic chemical substances, causing permanent health damage, contrary to the Hippocratic Oath. According to Bräutigam, the physician's duty to care for the patient's health and do no harm must supersede any government order.

The athletes who are present at the hearing, ready to testify against the duo are: Birgit Matz, Andrea Pinske, Jane Lang, Birgit Meineke-Heukrodt, Kerstin Olm, Carola Nitschke-Beraktschjan, Heike Meyer, Christiane Sommer and Marina Mende.

Here, we are going to see some of the most significant statements at the Binus–Gläser trial. The first is that of Berlinese swimmer Birgit Meineke-Heukrodt.

Like many athletes of her generation, she started her swimming career, back in 1974, at the prominent SC Dynamo Berlin. Initially, her results weren't very good, to the point that she failed to qualify for the Moscow Olympics; but everything changed when she was moved to Rolf Gläser's group. Gläser was one of the club's best coaches and under his supervision, Birgit Meineke improved her performances dramatically, becoming one of the fastest 100m freestyle swimmers, winning gold medals at the World Championships in Guayaquil (1982) and the European Championships in Rome (1983). With victories also came privileges: at 20 she was given her own flat and a Wartburg car. Meineke describes very positively the relationship she had with her coach: she considered Gläser a 'second father', until the day she found out about the real content of the 'cocktail' she would get from him. 'We would take "vitamins" dissolved in tea daily,' recalls the athlete, 'together with some injections. I can't understand how I was so gullible: pills and injections were an important factor that contributed to my victories, other than my training. I trusted my coaches blindly; how could I suspect that they were drugging me?'

Meineke underlines how certain explanations given to her by the doctors were surreal: 'When I noticed a change in my body's structure and my voice, they told me they were due to the swimming pool humidity. When I asked Dr Kipke why I had all those bouts of acne all over my body, he replied that it was down to the fact we girls didn't have enough sex!'[80]

In 1984, Birgit gave up sport to pursue a career in medicine, becoming a surgeon a few years later. That's how she found out the anomalies in her body were caused by anabolic steroids. She also discovered that all the possible side effects (kidney and pancreatic dysfunctions, heart problems, etc) had been known about since the sixties. The sports club's doctors could not have been unaware of that information. Meineke lives today with many ailments, including liver cancer. Although she is happy to have testified and faced her demons, she is disillusioned about the outcome of the trial: 'I know how things go in the medicine world. Doctors will be fined but will avoid jail and their mentality will never change.'[81]

Unlike Birgit Meineke and other athletes, Carola Nitschke-Beraktschjan, former 100m breaststroke world record holder, had actually suspected, at some point, the real nature of the mysterious 'supportive means' and tried to resist them, without success. In the late 70s, Carola's phenomenal results

---

80   Karin Helmstaedt, *Fear of the future*, Alexandria Master Swimming website, 2009.
81   Steven Ungerleider, *Faust's Gold: Inside The East German Doping Machine*, St Martin's Press, 2013.

and a 20kg increase in her body mass alerted her parents, who warned her about the possibility that illicit substances might be circulating at the sports club. The young swimmer from Berlin pretended to ingest the pills, spitting them out. When Rolf Gläser found this out, he expelled her from the elite team, relegating her to the lower squad. Nitschke was later summoned by some *Stasi* officers, who tried to convince her to take the Oral-Turinabol, but she kept refusing. With time, her swimming performances got slower and slower to the point that she decided to retire right before the Moscow Olympics. Fortunately, Carola didn't suffer any of the physiological consequences which affect other athletes: her stubbornness in refusing to take drugs has probably preserved her health. She still decided to testify in favour of her former, and less lucky, colleagues. At the trial, in order to highlight the futility and danger of doping, the former swimmer delivers a powerful and unexpected statement to the judge: 'I am giving up my medals, my world records ... they were tainted, rotten symbols of a toxic society. I don't want them in my closet. I will send them to the FINA. The medals belong to those who were clean, who competed drug-free. ... If I were an American, I would feel cheated.'[82]

The outstanding sincerity of the former champion helps convince the judge and the jury that the *Dopingprozess* is not just a matter of crime but is also a big moral issue. The defendants' actions have to be considered in this light as well.

Christiane Knacke-Sommer came from a small town near Dresden. In 1975, when she was 13, she was admitted to the prestigious SC Dynamo Berlin, after showing a promising talent for swimming butterfly. The first years were difficult as young Christiane had to live far away from home and her

---

82   (abridged version) Steven Ungerleider, *Faust's Gold: Inside The East German Doping Machine*, St Martin's Press, 2013.

parents; Dieter Binus and Rolf Gläser made her feel welcome and took good care of her. Under them, the swimmer was able to join the Olympic team in a few years.

When she is called to testify, Knacke-Sommer says all the girls at the club were given blue pills regularly, in four-week cycles; Rolf Gläser supervised the distribution and made sure the athletes actually swallowed them: 'I didn't pay much attention to them, they had told us they were nutritional supplements and they wanted to be sure we didn't forget to take them.'[83]

After just two cycles of 'treatment', Christiane felt her body change and she started to achieve surprising results. In preparation for the 1977 European Championships in Sweden, she was also given a pink pill to be taken in cycles together with the blue pill. Her performance in the 100m butterfly was so good that she won the silver medal, right behind the Montréal '76 sensation Andrea Pollack. Just a week later, Knacke-Sommer set a new world record during a national event, becoming the first woman to swim 100m in under a minute.

Christiane began to observe extensive collateral effects on her body: sudden hair growth, a rough (typically masculine) voice and an uncontrollable increase in her libido. These undesirable consequences increased even more when, a year later, she got injections of Depot-Turinabol, a different type of steroid, and Pervitin, a methamphetamine which causes addiction. The use of the latter sparked a row between the high-ranking officials, Manfred Ewald and Manfred Höppner on one side, and Dieter Binus and his colleague Bernd Pansold on the other. Ewald and Höppner believed that Pervitin had to be eliminated from the doping list as it was deemed too dangerous; Binus and Pensold used

---

83 Frank Bachner, *In Der Ddr-Dopingpraxis 1st Eine Neue Ebene Erreicht: Mit Suchtmitteln zum Weltrekord*, Der Tagesspiegel, 8 August 1998.

it anyway. As a consequence, it was decided to increase the internal doping tests for swimmers in order to make sure doctors and trainers weren't using that drug. Even in the ruthless world of East German sport there had to be boundaries.[84]

When, at the trial, the attorney asks Christiane if she was ever told by Dr Binus and her coach Gläser that she had been given testosterone pills, her answer is clear: 'Never! They told us that both pills and injections were vitamins. We didn't know anything of their origin, but even if we did, we couldn't refuse them. There was a motto circulating among us: "Take the pill or die." These substances have destroyed me, both physically and mentally.' At this point, Knacke-Sommer's testimony gets more emotional. After poking around nervously in her bag, she forcefully throws the bronze medal she won at the Moscow Olympics: 'It's tainted, poisoned with drugs and a corrupt system. It is worthless and a terrible embarrassment to all Germans.'[85]

Andrea Pollack also testifies at the trial, confirming that swimmers were given tablets and injections. After retiring, Pollack would go on to work as a sports physiotherapist. The three-time Olympic gold medallist from Schwerin will die of cancer in 2019, aged only 57.[86]

A few years earlier, in 1989, in an interview with *Stern* magazine, Christiane Knacke-Sommer had been the first East German athlete to confess to competing with the help of doping. At the end of the trial, Knacke-Sommer, Andrea Pollack and Carola Nitschke all return their medals to FINA

---

84 Frank Bachner, *In Der Ddr-Dopingpraxis Ist Eine Neue Ebene Erreicht: Mit Suchtmitteln Zum Weltrekord*, Der Tagesspiegel, 8 August 1998.

85 Steven Ungerleider, *Faust's Gold: Inside The East German Doping Machine*, St Martin's Press, 2013.

86 *Trauer um Schwimmerin Olympiasiegerin Andrea Pollack gestorben*, Der Tagesspiegel, 15 March 2019.

and ask for their names to be removed from all official records. Their request is completely ignored.

Sylvia Gerasch's testimony is more delicate than that of other colleagues: in fact, the swimmer from Cottbus is one of the very few people who decide to bear witness whilst still an active athlete. After competing for SC Dynamo Berlin and the GDR, she is now with the united Germany team. Her presence attracts a lot of journalists. Gerasch's name appears in the *Stasi* files as an athlete who has benefited from doping substances; the press would like to know, among other things, if her win at the recent World Championships in Perth (1998) can be considered clean or not.

The swimmer's statement is particularly blunt: 'I think that if some athletes have suffered physical damage, they should be compensated: they really have to come forward and speak out about their condition. However, it is important that a correlation between doping and damage is 100 per cent proven. I believe it's not fair the press depicts all East German athletes as bad people, as if in the rest of the world nobody else took drugs. Yes, it's true, Dieter Lindemann, my trainer used to give me blue and pink pills; he told me they were good for my teeth! But I would spit them out. I suspected they were trying to give us illicit substances, but I wanted to compete without them.'[87]

Some members of FINA will criticise her as, according to their rules, she should have reported any suspicious doping attempt.

Gerasch's testimony adds another nail in the coffin of the two defendants. On 31 August 1998, Dr Binus is fined 9,000 marks, whilst Gläser gets away with 7,200. Just like other top East German officers, they both manage to avoid imprisonment.

---

87   Ludwig Mascolo, *Das ist gut für die Zähne*, Der Spiegel N.34, 1997.

Dorit Rösler and Ulrich Sünder

On a sticky and hot mid-August morning in 1998, the hearing schedule brings forward the first woman involved in the state-sponsored doping scheme: sports doctor Dorit Rösler. With appreciable precision, Dr Rösler tells of her experience within the system without the usual reticence that characterises other defendants' statements. Her declarations are very honest: 'It's all true! We gave them Oral-Turinabol. We recorded everything on paper: dates, pills, training regime.' Dorit Rösler's words are carefully weighed: she is literally confessing, in tears. Whilst she speaks to Judge Jurgen Warnatsch, she looks at Karen König, a double European champion freestyle swimmer, the only athlete present in the courtroom that day: 'I can only say that I am really sorry. I should have shown more courage. In Nazi Germany we did what we were told to do. The GDR doping machine was no different; we were just carrying out medical orders ... have we not learned anything?'[88] At that point, Karen König asks her if she would have given the same treatment to her children; the doctor replies: 'I have always asked myself the same question. I think in that period, in the East, I would have done it. We were all under pressure from the government. We had to produce winners ...' Those are Rösler's last words before she starts to weep bitterly.[89]

After abandoning her sports career, Karen König decided to pursue humanities studies, earning a degree in literature. The former swimmer tells the judge about the oppressive regime that permeated the sports club she attended: 'Pills and fear were our diet. My voice became so low and rough that when I answered the phone, people would mistake me for my

88   Craig Lord, *GDR 30 Years On: The Day In 1989 The Berlin Wall Came Tumbling Down On Doping Regime*, Swimming World Magazine, 9 November 2019.

89   (Abridged version) Steven Ungerleider, *Faust's Gold: Inside The East German Doping Machine*, St Martin's Press, 2013.

brother. I was also suffering from anxiety and depression. I couldn't get any help. The drugs they gave me made me really nervous; I was one step away from ending up in an asylum.'[90]

Karen König had been one of the first athletes to openly talk about the doping issue in an article she wrote for *Der Spiegel*: 'When I decided to retire from swimming, my coaches were really upset. I was discharged with dishonour. During my sports career I had accumulated a lot of money, about 30,000 marks. These were kept in a special account managed by the DTSB, and I could access it only at the end of my career. Because of the way I left, they confiscated my money and I never got it. ... Years later, I came to know about the steroids by Klaus Klemenz, one of my trainers. We met at Nikolaiviertel, in Berlin, with other former swimmers, a reunion after the fall of the Wall. On that occasion, during our conversation, I confessed that I would have liked to go back to race. Klemenz said that he could have helped me because he still had some 'blue pills'. I asked for an explanation and he admitted candidly that we were all given steroids. He even bragged about the fact that we never realised what we were taking! "What a pig!" was the only thought I had in that moment.'[91]

The hearing of Ulrich Sünder, supervisor of doping plan operations for the DSSV, the swimming federation, since 1971, begins a few hours after Dorit Rösler's. Sünder's position was that of a typical bureaucrat, in charge of tasks that would allow him to 'pass the buck' and assign blame to other people. His words are quite sharp: 'The word "doping" didn't even exist, at that time. The term we used was *"Unterstützende Mittel"* (supportive means) – it looked more appropriate. Some of our athletes knew the origin of the substances they took, but as long as they won, everything was fine. Others, on the other hand, didn't train properly, didn't race properly and their bodies

---

90   Ibid.

91   Karen König, *'Warum lügen alle?'*, Der Spiegel, 25 April 1994.

didn't tolerate the drugs; I think these athletes have developed a certain form of resentment towards the sport system. Even some parents knew that their children took drugs, but they looked the other way, as long as they won medals and enjoyed the bonuses. I knew about the virilising effect on women, but I had been told that the effects were temporary and that their bodies would return to normal once stopping the taking of Oral-Turinabol. You have to understand that during the Honecker regime, sport was part of politics, and whoever had connections with that world might get certain privileges which were out of reach for other East German citizens. It was difficult to give them up.'[92]

After the hearing, it only takes a couple of days for the verdict to be decided by Judge Warnatsch. The two East German officers are sentenced to pay a fine of a few thousand marks, and they avoid imprisonment. Again, a light punishment but, this time, the trial has confirmed, through some important confessions, the existence of a state doping plan and that many athletes are still suffering physiological and psychological stress because of it.[93]

At the end of the verdict reading, Dorit Rösler approaches Karen König and tries to shake her hand. The former swimmer hesitates for a few seconds but then decides to accept Rösler's apology. König asks the doctor if she could help her to shed some light on those dark years and bring more officers to justice. Karen König will take the NOK (the German Olympic Committee) to court in 2005 and, thanks to Dorit Rösler's testimony, she will be given 10,200 euros in compensation.[94]

The convictions handed down by the Berlinese judges represent a small moral victory for the athletes. Unfortunately,

92 Interviewed in the TV documentary *Doping for Gold*, PBS, 2007.
93 Edmund L. Andrews, *3 Guilty of Giving Drugs To East German Athletes*, The New York Times, 21 August 1998.
94 Kate Connolly, *East German swimming star sues over drug scandal*, The Telegraph, 2 November 2005.

as predicted by the defence lawyers, all the coaches and doctors implicated in the system got away with paying fines, keeping in most cases their professional licences, their careers and even gaining some fame as TV pundits.

5.

DOPINGPROZESS: ACT II

AS WE have seen, the first two years of the state-sponsored doping trials end with some suspended jail sentences. Defendants (doctors, managers and coaches) get away with just fines: none of them go to prison. None of the political members of the SED or the government are called to testify in the courtroom.

Judge Bräutigam tries to explain the reason behind those decisions: 'The sentences are not very heavy because the defendants were accused of violating the law of a nation that doesn't exist anymore. Legally, we were moving in uncharted territory and we had to be very careful. Our intention was to be lenient with the "corporals" and harsh with the "generals", but we couldn't bring to the dock any of the political bosses of the former GDR.'[95]

Despite the laughable penalties, a positive outcome materialises in the form of a new law passed by the *Bundestag*, which establishes a ten-year jail term for anyone who gives steroids to underage children. Another useful result is the acknowledgement that many athletes had suffered damage to their health because of the state-sponsored doping programme, entitling them to some form of compensation.

---

95 Steven Ungerleider, *Faust's Gold: Inside The East German Doping Machine*, St Martin's Press, 2013.

In 2000, all defendants appeal the court's decisions but their pleas are rejected by the *Bundesgerichtshof,* the German Supreme Court.

The Two Manfreds

In the same year, on 2 May 2000, the final part of the trial begins. Manfred Höppner and Manfred Ewald are in the dock: the former was a high-level sports doctor and deputy head of the Sports Medicine Service; the latter was president of the German Gymnastic and Sports Federation (DTSB) and chairman of the Olympic Committee. The hearing is chaired by Judge Dirk Dickhaus; the charges against them come from 142 athletes! Among these sportsmen and sportswomen, there are famous and less prominent names from East German swimming and athletics, like Rica Reinisch, Karen König, Martina Gottschalt, Ute Krause, Jutta Gottschalk, Birgit Matz, Carola Nitschke-Beraktschjan, Birgit Heukrodt, Kornelia Otto, Kornelia Ender, Andreas Krieger, Michael Dröse, Margitta Pufe, Barbara Krause, Petra Schneider, Christiane Knacke-Sommer, Catherine Menschner, Kathleen Nord, Ines Geipel, Birgit Paist Boese, Yvonne Stierwald Bebhardt, Marita Koch, Simone Michel Machalett, Brigitte Sander Michel and Martina Opitz Hellman.

Manfred Höppner was the real leader and coordinator of the state-sponsored doping programme in the GDR. His supervisory 'debut' at the Olympics in 1968 coincided with shot putter Margitta Gummel's exploits, when, as we have seen, she won the gold medal after being subjected to the first massive anabolic steroid programme.

Höppner can be described as a sort of Dr Jekyll and Mr Hyde, a powerful bureaucrat with a 'split personality': whilst on the one hand he devised and implemented the doping plan, on the other, as an IAAF member, he presented himself as a bold doping opponent.[96]

---

96 Steven Ungerleider, Faust's Gold: Inside the East German Doping Machine, St Martin's Press, 2013.

Before the start of the hearing, Judge Dickhaus allows the defendant to read a statement. The tone of his speech is self-justifying, almost surreal, and makes the other people present in the courtroom, especially the former athletes, upset.

'Competitive sport begins where healthy sport ends. Where is the difference between sport and the real world? ... Many people take drugs in order to maintain their capacity to work efficiently.'

Höppner essentially speculates about the legitimacy of the athletes taking drugs in order to perform properly in their jobs. 'The use of drugs includes the prevention of damage. We carried out scientific studies to prove that it was possible to use the "supportive means" to enhance performance, without causing any damage. Our main objective was to minimise injury and maximise training hours.'[97]

The audience present in the courtroom begins to rumble: the former athletes feel mocked by Höppner's words. However, in spite of the passionate 'moral defence' of his work, the court decided that he was responsible for implementing the state-sponsored doping plan and pushing the administration of steroids to underage athletes without their consent. There is enough evidence for a severe punishment.

A few days later, it's Manfred Ewald's turn. His line of defence is one of total denial. Ewald (a former Nazi) decides to adopt a reticent stance; he rejects all accusations, claiming to be morally innocent, denying any involvement with the state-sponsored doping. At this point, Judge Dickhaus, having ascertained the non-cooperative attitude of the defendant, decides to hear some of the witnesses' stories. Let's see the most significant.

Swimmer Carola Nitschke-Beraktschjan reveals she was first given steroids in pills when she was 11. The former 100m

---

97   (Abridged version) Steven Ungerleider, *Faust's Gold: Inside the East German Doping Machine*, St Martin's Press, 2013.

breaststroke world record holder reveals that, by the time she was 14, she would be given 30 pills a day![98] At some point, they started to give her injections: 'They would do them in my bottom. When I asked them what medicine was that, they got angry. After a while, my voice became rough and masculine; when I asked for an explanation, they told me dismissively not to worry about it: I had to swim, not to sing, after all!'[99]

The tension in the courtroom builds up quite dramatically when it's Ute Krause's turn. The former swimmer from Berlin describes with great accuracy her training, the endless physiological tests, the 'vitamin drinks', and the coloured pills she was given. She also vividly illustrates the weird changes to her body and how this eventually led to an eating disorder and her leaving the sport.[100] Krause accuses Höppner and Ewald of ruining her life when she attended the sports club. Her main problems were depression, bulimia and anorexia; these were so serious that she was forced to give up her place at the Moscow Olympics: 'I was always ill but the doctors kept telling me to take the pills. I didn't understand what was happening to me and I didn't know who to ask for help. I couldn't trust anyone. One day I passed out and I woke up in a pool of my own vomit; that was the sign that I had to stop.'[101] The promising athlete decided to abandon all sports to recover and take care of her health.

Years later, in 1984, Ute Krause got a job as a carer in a nursing home. At some point, one of the people she was attending had to take some drugs, which looked very familiar:

98 *Germany's solution to drug stain just won't wash*, The Sydney Morning Herald, 2 April 2003.

99 Jürgen Holz, *Ewald schweigt weiter*, Neuse Deutschland, 20 May 2000.

100 Domnhall Macauley, *Doping in sport – a warning from history*, British Medical Journal, 22 September 2007.

101 Steven Ungerleider, *Faust's Gold: Inside The East German Doping Machine*, St Martin's Press, 2013.

pink and blue pills, the same type she had seen years before at the sports club. The only difference, this time, was that she could read the information leaflet included within the box. The name of the drug was Oral-Turinabol. Ute ran frantically to her supervisor, a doctor, to ask what the drugs were for. The physician explained that they were an anabolic steroid used to treat cancer patients to boost their immune system.[102] He also added, knowing that Krause was a former swimmer, that those chemicals were used to improve athletes' performances. The revelation was, of course, quite shocking, but at that time there was very little to do; she couldn't tell anyone without facing the consequences.[103]

Obviously, Höppner and Ewald try to defend themselves, attempting to convince (without success) the judge that, in spite of their involvement in the state-sponsored doping programme, they were just gears in the medal-producing machine. Their lawyer, Hans Peter Mildebrandt, tries to minimise (and, at times, ridicule) the drugs' nasty consequences on the athletes' health, questioning the correlation between steroids and illness. Judge Dickhaus is not impressed.

Giving evidence, Rica Reinisch, the three-time Olympic champion, lets out all her frustration at Mildebrandt's provocation: 'You really don't want to listen! I am constantly in pain. My ovaries are always inflamed; I had two miscarriages and I have to take beta blockers regularly because of a cardiac arrhythmia, but you don't care.'[104]

Young Rica's problems had started during a tour of competitions in Russia: 'It was awful. All of a sudden I got severe belly cramps. I didn't know what was going on. When I returned to East Germany, my parents took me to a doctor

---

102 Nowadays, anabolic steroids are no longer prescribed for this purpose. Modern medicine prefers to use corticosteroids.

103 Steven Ungerleider, *Faust's Gold: Inside The East German Doping Machine*, St Martin's Press, 2013.

104 Interview in the documentary *Doping for Gold*, PBS, 2007.

who found some ovarian cysts. In that moment, I realised that the pills they gave me had had a negative effect on my health. In addition, I noticed the unexpected growth of unwanted hair and my voice became deeper. I tried to ask the other swimmers to see if they were experiencing similar problems, but nobody wanted to talk about it. The underage swimmers didn't know what was going on, but the young adults did. Some colleagues of mine used to say: 'Why do you complain? If the pills make you go faster and win … Don't you want to win?' I was very confused; I didn't know what to do. When my parents found out they were giving me drugs, they went mad. I remember my mother came to pick me up at Sport Club Einheit Dresden and shouted at my coach, Uwe Neumann, in front of everybody else, saying that he should never try to see me again. That was my last day in a swimming pool.'[105]

Rica Reinisch's former sports club has a hall of fame, a corridor with giant pictures of distinguished swimmers. Even today, the section where Rica's picture was is empty. This shows that, even many years after the fall of the Berlin Wall, her retirement was seen as a betrayal by the club's managers, who implemented a sort of *damnatio memoriae* to athletes who went against the system. The sportswoman from Saxony wonders how the defendants could sacrifice the East German teenagers' lives just to win medals. Reinisch's last statement is particularly bitter and shows all her disillusionment: 'We were just "diplomats in tracksuits". The worst thing they did was to take away from me the opportunity to ever know if I could have won the gold medals without the steroids.'[106]

Rica Reinisch's words are followed by declarations of similar tone and significance from Karen König, Heike

---

105 Interview in the documentary *Doping for Gold*, PBS, 2007. A very similar scene to this episode features in the German TV Series, *Der gleiche Himmel* (The Same Sky, 2017), broadcast on ZDF.

106 ABC NEWS, *20/20 East German Doping Scandal*, 13 October 2000.

Rödiger Grünler and Ines Geipel. The latter tells quite poignantly how the *Stasi* ruined her sports career as they suspected she might consider defecting to a Western country. During a training session in Mexico, young Ines befriended a Mexican athlete and had confessed to her parents she wanted to leave East Germany. Once back in her country, her club's doctors convinced her to have her appendix removed, to improve her performances, but it was just an excuse to cut through her abdomen's muscles: that operation ended her career and, above all, curbed any craving to leave the country. The most disturbing aspect of this account, tragic enough in itself, is that the person who revealed Ines's plans to the authorities was her father, a particularly zealous *Stasi* agent. A rather chilling note on a declassified document states: 'Now we have finally found an opportunity to put her on ice.'[107]

'Particularly zealous' is a label that can also be attached to Heinz Ender, father of swimming sensation Kornelia, winner of four gold medals at the 1976 Olympic Games in Montréal. One year later, when the athlete suspected she had been given steroids, she decided to leave her club, SV Halle, and go to study medical sciences to become a physiotherapist. In the summer of 1989, Kornelia tried to flee to West Germany with her family, via Hungary and Austria, but the Hungarian police, alerted by a trusted source, arrested her. Once back in East Germany, the swimmer found out that the 'trusted source' was her father, an army colonel. Fortunately, the events surrounding the fall of the Berlin Wall would spare her a lengthy imprisonment.[108] Today, Kornelia Ender works as a physiotherapist in a small town near Mainz and, happily, she has never experienced any doping-related health issue.

---

107 Steve Scott, *The young athletes whose lives were shattered by a secret doping programme in East Germany*, documentary, ITV (UK), broadcast 25 May 2017.

108 Erik Eggers and Detlef Hacke, *Honeckers Porzellan*, Der Spiegel, 10 January 2015.

On 30 May 2000, Judge Dickhaus, former athletes and members of the press, attend one of the most emotional and moving hearings: Andreas Krieger's. At the European Athletics Championships in Stuttgart, in 1986, shot putter Heidi Krieger attained the best result of her career: a gold medal, thanks to a 21.10m throw. Today, Andreas is Heidi's *alter ego*. The accretion of steroids in her body resulted in a devastating cumulative effect, to the point that Heidi started to feel more and more like a man, not only chemically but also psychologically. After many years of identity crisis, Heidi decided to become Andreas. Werner Franke underlines that the amount of steroids in Krieger's body surpassed that taken by Canadian sprinter Ben Johnson: 'With all those pills, it was inevitable that masculine developments were permanent.'[109]

Before starting the hearing, Andreas asks Judge Dickhaus if he might approach the bench to show him a piece of paper; the judge assents. Dickhaus, with great interest, unfolds the paper and looks at a picture of Andreas, or actually Heidi, as a young athlete. Andreas adds: 'I wanted you to see me when I was a girl, your Honour. I wanted you to see me how I was before they started to pump me with drugs and assault me with psychological violence. Before they unleashed the hell that made me change sex.'[110]

Andreas tries to explain the dreadful atmosphere at SC Dynamo Berlin: 'To give you an idea, one day I was in a hospital because of severe cramps; Dr Windler came to see me, but instead of taking care of my health, he ordered me to get up from the bed and get ready for a competition. We athletes were treated like machines. ... My relationship with people was awful. I couldn't go around. I didn't feel like a woman anymore: I looked like a man and the others were making fun

---

109 Interview in the documentary *Doping for Gold*, PBS, 2007.
110 Steven Ungerleider, *Faust's Gold: Inside The East German Doping Machine*, St Martin's Press, 2013.

of me: they would call me "transvestite". I preferred to remain inside the school, shielded from the outside world. I asked for help, but the doctors ignored me. I wanted to kill myself. Finally, in 1997, I realised who I had become and I managed to get an operation and change sex officially. I feel better now, but I am always depressed and I am unemployed. Fortunately, my mother helped me a lot. Dr Höppner certainly had some files about me, but he has presumably destroyed them to hide my illness.'[111]

At the end of the hearing, Andreas Krieger confirms he intends to send his medals back to the IAAF. In 2002, he marries former swimmer Ute Krause; the two met during the trial. Today, Andreas runs a military memorabilia shop in Magdeburg.

Other athletes are heard by Judge Dickhaus but the tone of their accounts doesn't differ much from those he has seen before. After two and a half months, Dickhaus has collected enough evidence and he is ready to deliver his verdict. On 18 July 2000, Manfred Ewald and Manfred Höppner are convicted 'as accessories to intentional bodily harm of athletes, including minors', handed a two-year prison term (suspended) and ordered to pay 'the costs (10,000 marks) of the proceedings and those of the 20 co-plaintiffs'.[112] Whilst Dr Höppner eventually apologises for any harm caused, Ewald has never shown any remorse; his lawyer, Frank Osterloh, tries desperately, but in vain, to convince the judge that there was no guilt at all under the GDR law. In 2001, both their sentences are confirmed by the Federal Court.[113]

In his final speech, Judge Dickhaus explains that the real objective of the trial has never been to judge the contradictions

---

111 Documentary *Heidi's Farthest Throw*, available on andreas-krieger-story.org/.

112 *'Es ist erst mal gut'*, Der Spiegel, 18 July 2000.

113 Federal Court of Justice decision of 5 September 2001 in the criminal case against Manfred Ewald.

of the East German political system, but to punish the offences. The most important aspect to consider is that, in the GDR, doping wasn't even considered a crime, therefore the only valid accusatory element was based on violation of human rights: the fact that the defendants voluntarily distributed doping substances to about 10,000 underage athletes. Officials, doctors and coaches knew about the physiological damage that the drugs would cause. This awareness didn't stop them from administering them anyway. The end couldn't justify the means.[114]

Despite the leniency of the sentencing, all the convictions from the three-year-long trial have the merit of defining an important principle: the fact that many GDR athletes are now acknowledged as victims of the state-sponsored doping system, and not partners in crime, and, as such, they could be entitled to compensation or some form of financial support. As we'll explore in the following chapters, this help will materialise in the form of a series of controversial one-off payments decided, from time to time, by the parliament.

At the end of the *prozess*, all the former athletes show some relief and a deep sense of gratitude towards Werner Franke, Brigitte Berendonk and Michael Lehner, without whom the trial would never have had a chance to start. In 2004, for their continuous and remarkable effort in search of the truth, Werner Franke and Brigitte Berendonk are awarded the highest federal decoration, *Verdienstorden der Bundesrepublik Deutschland*, the Order of Merit of the Federal Republic of Germany.[115]

114 Steven Ungerleider, *Faust's Gold: Inside The East German Doping Machine*, St Martin's Press, 2013.
115 Doping-Opfer-Hilfe website.

6.

THE MANY SIDES OF A MEDAL

IN THIS dramatic story of physiological and psychological abuse perpetrated on young athletes, we have seen a fairly common reaction from the victims: they loudly condemned the state-sponsored doping in East Germany and, in some cases, relinquished their victories and returned their medals, in order to underline the principle of distancing themselves from a corrupt and perverse system.

In this chapter we'll explore the behaviour of those sportsmen and sportswomen who, for whatever reason, did not attend the trial and who have had limited media exposure. Some are gold medal winners but some are also unknown athletes whose hopes of glory have faded into obscurity. We will also examine some lesser-known aspects of state doping: the drugs' long-term consequences, their psychological effects and how different athletes reacted to the oppressive system. All of them have a remarkable story to tell.

Deserved medals

Some athletes have never accepted the narrative inscribed on the secret documents found in the *Stasi* archives or the 'procedural truth' that emerged from the *Dopingprozess*; they are strongly convinced that their wins are due to years of hard training and are therefore fully deserved. To them, there is no reason to hide or throw away their medals, or be ashamed of having won them.

When, in 2005, former sprinter Ines Geipel asked the DLV, the German Athletics Association, to cancel her 4x100 relay world record (together with hundreds of other records set over 20 years by the GDR), her team-mates weren't impressed. Bärbel Wöckel, Marlies Göhr and Ingrid Auerswald showed great camaraderie towards their friend back in 1984, when she fled the training camp to secretly meet a Mexican athlete; now they don't even want to hear about Ines. Former 100m world record holder Göhr thinks Geipel is just someone looking for a moment of fame and her request to erase the records is nonsense: 'We made our country proud; I am not a victim and I am not an accuser. I am just a winner.[116] I can't believe that drugs can make you run faster. The only thing that counts is training.'[117]

The former runner insists she has never taken drugs, despite the fact that the *Stasi* files tell a different story: in 1984, at the top of their career, the four SC Motor Jena sprinters took the following amounts of Oral-Turinabol: Geipel, 1,291mg; Wöckel, 1,670mg; Auerswald, 1,375mg; Göhr, 1,405mg.[118] Ingrid Auerswald is adamant that their wins were due to hard training and placing such importance on the role of doping is absurd.[119] Bärbel Wöckel doesn't even want to talk about it: 'It all happened many years ago.' Another former champion, Marita Koch, has threatened to sue the DLV, should they decide to write her name off the list of world record holders.[120]

In 2006, the DLV agreed to substitute Ines Geipel's name with an asterisk in their record list. The same request was

---

116 Gerhard Pfeil, *Gegen die Nebelwand*, Der Spiegel, N.17, April2006.
117 Documentary *ABC Foreign Correspondent: For Greater Glory*, Australian Broadcasting Corporation, broadcast 16 August 2016.
118 Brigitte Berendonk, *Von der Forschung zum Betrug*, Springer Verlag, 1991.
119 Gerhard Pfeil, *Gegen die Nebelwand*, Der Spiegel, N.17, April2006.
120 Gerhard Pfeil, *Gegen die Nebelwand*, Der Spiegel, N.17, April 2006.

granted, four years later, to Gesine Walther, who had set a 4x400 world record, together with Marita Koch, Sabine Busch and Dagmar Rübsam, in 1984. After years of debate and legal discussions, the DLV decided not to cancel the old records, unless an athlete requests it. The official IAAF record lists still retain Geipel and Walther's names.

Whilst some athletes reasonably think that their medals were deserved because they had been achieved through hard training and shouldn't be questioned, other athletes have mixed views. While admitting the existence of the doping system, they claim the legitimacy of their wins. In a TV documentary produced by PBS, *Doping for Gold*, US swimmer Wendy Boglioli, who often came second behind the GDR athletes, goes to Berlin to visit Petra Thümer, who won a few races in her event. The American star asks her former rival how she considers her victories in light of the documented fact that all GDR athletes competed with the support of anabolic steroids. Thümer's reply is honest and straight: 'It's difficult to say. I was very young and I had no idea of the doping system and how widespread it was. However, I don't think it's fair to question my wins; they came thanks to hard work and many hours of training. My country made many mistakes, but I don't think it was the only one to distribute doping to its athletes.'[121]

Some athletes, like javelin thrower Ruth Fuchs, admit to have used doping substances knowingly ('I'm not one of those who say I didn't do that … a lot of money was involved')[122], without renouncing their medals. Fuchs was supported by Karl Hellmann, her husband and coach. At the end of her sports career, the athlete from Saxony switched to politics, becoming a member of parliament.

---

121 Documentary *Doping for Gold*, PBS, 2007.
122 Ruth Fuchs, *Bekennende Doping-Sportlerin*, Berliner Zeitung, 8 April 1994.

Former sprint legend Marita Koch – who ran distances from 100m to 400m with record-breaking times[123] – has always said she never took drugs. However, some evidence shows she may have been aware of performance-enhancing pills. In a letter, found in the *Stasi* archives, sent in 1986 to her coach, Michael Öttel, Koch allegedly complains about the low quality of the drugs she took: 'Mine are not as powerful as the ones you gave to Barbel Eckert, who keeps running faster than me.'[124] The athlete, however, has always cast doubts on the validity of the *Stasi* documents – we will discuss this controversial topic in Chapter 8.

Fourteen years later, Marita Koch attends the trial against Ewald and Höppner, where the truth about the doping system comes out; she will always oppose any decision to retroactively cancel her wins.[125]

Legendary sprinter and jumper Heike Drechsler also changes her approach to the 'supportive means' she had been given when she was at SC Motor Jena. After taking Brigitte Berendonk to court for slander in 1995, and losing her lawsuit, she accepts, in 2001, that she was a victim of the state-sponsored doping programme. Today, Drechsler is a well-known person in the German media and she is also engaged in promoting motivation and work/life balance.[126]

It is understandable that many athletes don't want their victories removed or tarnished; after all, regardless of doping (which was taken unknowingly in most cases), they worked hard to achieve their world record-breaking performances, and to them it is a matter of pride and moral conduct, that

---

123 Marita Koch is currently the 400m world record holder (47.60 seconds), set in Canberra, 6 October 1985.

124 Steven Ungerleider, *Faust's Gold: Inside The East German Doping Machine*, St Martin's Press, 2013 (Appendix 1).

125 Jutta Hees, *Zurück auf Start*, Taz, 22 March 2006.

126 Duncan Mackey, *Drechsler: 'I took drugs'*, The Guardian, 17 January 2001.

should be free from any technical or chemical interference. Imagine this: you train hard for several hours a day, for six days a week, for ten years; you have little or no social life, and spend a long time away from your family. You see your body change but you don't understand exactly why; you feel weird. Your friends live a normal teenage life but you can't: your homeland needs you. You can't even eat an ice cream when you would like to. Then, you win one or more medals; you bring glory to your country. All your sacrifices have been rewarded, but in 1998 they tell you that, because you had been given doping when you were 12 (and at 12 you didn't even know the difference between sugar and testosterone), you are a cheat, a liar. Give your medals back! It is only reasonable that an athlete who went through years of sacrifices might experience a moment of cognitive dissonance. It must seem incredibly unfair being treated like a fraud, after having been lied to by your own government. It is understandable that each former GDR athlete reacts in a different way, and it is equally understandable that those who have been defeated feel cheated and want to be compensated. There will be time to discuss this nearly philosophical concept in Chapter 8.

The IOC decided to adopt an eight-year 'statute of limitations' rule: any offence related to doping must be discovered within that period of time, starting from the day the transgression takes place. The IAAF and the FINA, in line with the IOC's policy, have confirmed that they have no intention of cancelling the old records.

The last gold in Montréal

In spite of the IOC's rigid stance, there is someone who hasn't given up hope of seeing a reassignment of the medals. Former US swimmer Shirley Babashoff, who came second four times behind the East German girls at the Olympics in Montréal '76, has always complained, publicly and rather emphatically, about the weird masculine appearance of those GDR athletes and, above all, their wins, deeming them unmerited and unfair. This attitude, however, only earned her the reputation of a bad loser – the American press nicknamed her 'Surly Shirley'. Babashoff used to get on the podium in tears, refusing to congratulate the winner; during a press conference, she even highlighted the physical differences between the two teams, implying that although the US lost the races, they at least looked like women.[127] The American swimmer was 100 per cent sure that their adversaries had cheated.

During the Olympics, the emotional state of the US swimmers was very low. The team trained very hard to reach the perfect athletic condition for the Games, but they couldn't win anymore and their coaches didn't understand why. Many American sports journalists accused them of being spoiled, of behaving like prima donnas and being unable to lose with dignity.

With every race in the women's programme having ended in disappointment – all won by Eastern Bloc athletes – the Americans had one last opportunity on the final day: the 4x100 freestyle relay. For the USA it was a matter of national pride: they must win. Previously, however, the GDR had won the 4x100 medley relay race, improving the world record by an amazing six seconds![128] All commentators, experts and insiders knew there was no hope for the US team. What they had seen up to this moment looked pretty clear: the East German swimming team was from a different planet and the American girls seemed too confused and disconcerted to focus properly on their last race. Another silver medal looked more than likely.

However, the American fans hoped that a rush of pride might inspire the US swimmers to go beyond expectations.

---

127 Doug Gilbert, *The Miracle Machine*, Coward, McCann & Geoghegan, 1980.

128 1) GDR (Richter, Anke, Ender, Pollack) 4:07.95, 2) USA (Jezek, Siering, Wright, Babashoff) 4:14.55, 3) Canada (Hogg, Corsiglia, Sloan, Jardin) 4:15.22.

The American girls were actually very much in the mood to perform a miracle, and the fact that the two teams swam next to each other (in lanes three and four), made the race even more interesting, as the swimmers could monitor their opponent's position more clearly. After a false start, the race began nervously and immediately got really exciting. GDR's Kornelia Ender's start was impressive: during her 100m she gained centimetre after centimetre on her US opponent, Kim Peyton; the girl from Oregon finished about 1.5m behind the East German – not the best start for the Americans, but Peyton's performance was still a good one.

The East Germans were used to increasing their advantage more and more as a relay progressed, but this time, during the second leg, an unexpected turnaround materialised at the Aquatic Centre as Wendy Boglioli succeeded in actually reducing the gap to about half a metre from Petra Priemer. During the third leg, Jill Sterkel incredibly managed to close the gap, completing her 100m alongside Andrea Pollack. After three-quarters of the relay, the two teams were level; all was now in the hands of Shirley Babashoff, racing against Claudia Hempel. Babashoff's determination was beyond measure; she knew her team-mates had worked a miracle to give her the chance for a final head-to-head dash with the East German athlete and she couldn't fail. And she didn't. Her last 50m was nothing short of a masterpiece. The first hand to touch the lane sensor was hers: gold medal for the USA, and a new world record.[129]

Among the hundreds of gold medals won by the USA in the history of the Olympic Games, that one, earned by the 4x100 freestyle team in Montréal is one of the most memorable and evocative, perhaps because it was one of the most difficult to achieve: won through sheer determination

---

129 1) USA (Peyton, Boglioli, Sterkel, Babashoff) 3:44.82, 2) GDR (Ender, Priemer, Pollack, Hempel) 3:45.50, 3) Canada (Amundrud, Clark, Smith, Jardin) 3:48.81.

against a phantom adversary, deemed impossible to beat by everyone. Despite the win, the American press and the fans didn't really appreciate the team's statements and behaviour after the race. As the East German girls tried to congratulate her on the podium, Shirley Babashoff ignored them and turned her back. She and her team-mates would keep accusing the East Germans of cheating, even several weeks after the event. As Wendy Boglioli recalls: 'I used to get death threats after I came back from the Olympics from all these people that would send me nasty letters, nasty messages on my phone about "how dare the American women accuse these poor East German women of taking steroids, they are just better than you, face it!"'[130]

In light of the discovery of the GDR state-sponsored doping plan, Shirley Babashoff has often pleaded the case of the redistribution of Olympic medals, and she would be pleased to meet the IOC's president to discuss her reasons: 'I would love that but I am afraid that he would just spew the eight-year rule at me. It was 13 years after the fact [referring to the East Germans] before we had proof. Why is there a statute of limitations? It is just dumb. It is like trying to talk to a crazy person. Who knows how the IOC thinks? There are probably some people in the IOC who don't even know swimming.'[131]

However, not all her team-mates share her view; Jill Sterkel thinks that 'what happened to the East German girls is horrible. I don't ask to take their medals away; I believe they already suffered enough. I am lucky to be born in America.'[132] Jack Nelson, the girls' coach, has provocatively suggested that the American Olympic Committee present its athletes

---

130 Interview in *The Perfect Race, 20/20*, by Elizabeth Vargas, produced by Barbara Walters and Janice Tomlin, ABC TV, October 2000.

131 Swimming World Magazine, Brent Rutemiller, *Shirley Babashoff wants her place in history*, 15 September, 2016.

132 Interview in the documentary *The Last Gold* (Brian T. Brown, 2016).

with gold medal copies, as a symbolic gesture. Nelson has always complained about the fact that, in spite of the many prestigious medals won by Babashoff and her team-mates, the press and the world of sports generally had unfairly snubbed their achievements.[133]

In 2016, after a few animated interviews released by Shirley Babashoff, the Senate of California decided to formally ask the IOC to reconsider the possibility of redistributing the Montréal '76 medals to more deserving athletes.

A few years earlier, symbolically, the magazine *Swimming World* had decided to remove all East German athletes who were elected 'Swimmer of the Year', criticising the IOC for not considering the topic of the redistribution of medals even worth a discussion.[134] In 2016, the magazine's publishers presented the International Swimming Federation (FINA) with a list of proposals to right the wrongs, with a few intriguing twists. Here is an extract from the plea:

> ... Almost everyone agreed that the systematic doping of athletes by the East German government affected the Olympics medal standings. Swimming World acknowledged that the GDR women were just as much victims as were the swimmers who were cheated out of winning medals and their place in history. ... On behalf of the swimming community worldwide, we are calling on FINA to recognise all victims during this dark period in Olympic history and to lobby the International Olympic Committee to take similar action.
>
> We therefore ask the following:

---

133 Brent Rutemiller, Swimming World, *1976 US Olympic Head Coach Jack Nelson Tells Emotional Tale of Montreal*, 28 November 2013.

134 Swimming World, *Stripped! Swimming World Vacates Awards of GDR Drug-Fueled Swimmers*, 1 December 2013.

1. That FINA acknowledge that the aquatic records were tainted during the GDR era.

2. That FINA acknowledge that there were victims on both sides of the podium.

3. That FINA place an asterisk next to all GDR era swimmers, explaining that they were unknowingly doped.

4. That FINA acknowledge a second tier of new medal standings (consisting of those not recognised) alongside the existing standings of GDR victims.

5. That FINA not ask for GDR swimmers to return their medals.

6. That FINA award duplicate medals to those athletes who have a new standing.

7. That FINA remove from its list of Pin winners all GDR officials, including the convicted Dr Lothar Kipke, a former Medical Commission delegate who was found guilty of harm to minors in the German doping trials of the late 1990s.

8. That FINA stage an event where those who are affected by the reordering of the medals meet with the GDR women in a spirit of sportsmanship, consolation, and forgiveness.

The final request above could be the most impactful for all parties and victims. We cannot think of anything more powerful, emotional and meaningful than FINA staging a medal ceremony during the World Championships. A ceremony of this nature speaks to all that is good about forgiveness, sportsmanship and above all the spirit of humanity.[135]

---

135 Swimming World Magazine, *An Open Letter Asking FINA To Recognise All Victims During The DDR Olympic Reign*, 28 April 2016.

The open letter was also published as a petition on the famous portal *change.org*, collecting only 1,513 supporters. It almost goes without saying that *Swimming World*'s open letter has been largely ignored.

Long-term consequences

Petra Thümer, Ruth Fuchs, Heike Drechsler and many other East German athletes have been lucky enough not to suffer any permanent physical damage from the intake of anabolic steroids. In fact, not all people subject to the doping programme have developed the typical health problems linked to high levels of testosterone we have seen in the previous chapters. The assimilation of certain drugs doesn't necessarily cause the onset of medical conditions, but it certainly increases the risk of them happening to people who are genetically predisposed.

Scientists have recently tried to explore correlations between steroids and ailments, and to what extent the second is triggered by the first. Former swimmer and surgeon Sigurd Hanke, a self-confessed doper, confirms how hard it is to find a definite relationship and that other factors should be taken into account: 'From a medical point of view, it is difficult today to separate the health consequences of doping from a normal, fateful course of life, and it becomes more and more difficult the longer the doping practice has been in the past. In addition, there is hardly any data on many of the substances used, and certainly not on possible side effects or even late effects. Finding out such connections is already difficult with normal approved medicines. A distinction must also be made between primary, i.e. immediate consequences of the doping substances, and secondary consequences of excessive training, missing breaks in the event of illness, and reduced pain perception which was made possible by the doping substances. And last but not least, there is also physical and mental damage from excessively practised sport alone, i.e.

without taking any drugs. Anything overdone is unhealthy. This also includes high-performance sport.'[136]

It looks clear that establishing a proven connection between chemistry and illness is not an easy task. Nevertheless, there have been a few important attempts.

In a study conducted in 2012 by Dr Giselher Spitzer on a sample of 50 former GDR athletes, it emerges that 25 per cent of them have developed serious cardiac and liver problems, and 10 per cent have cancer. Some have also suffered from depression and self-harm tendencies. Most women have experienced miscarriage.[137]

According to Spitzer's evaluation, these results are very high compared to the average population, a sign that a correlation between the intake of testosterone and certain disorders might exist. In fairness, a 50-athlete sample doesn't appear to be enormously significant, but it certainly provides an important input to study this phenomenon further. Professor Harald Freyberger, a leading psychiatrist at the Ernst-Moritz-Arndt University of Greifswald, monitored for many years the long-term effects of doping substances. In 2017 he published his study, showing the shocking result that doped athletes from the GDR live, on average, 10–12 years less than 'normal people', and that the probability they get seriously ill is 2.7 times higher (3.2 in the case of mental illness).[138] Freyberger's research also shows that former athletes mainly suffer depression and eating disorders.

Many of these athletes are not even known to the public as they never took part in major sports tournaments and never won anything significant. One of them, discus thrower Katja Hofmann, has recently decided to tell of her experience,

136 Correspondence with the author.
137 Giselher Spitzer, *Doping in der DDR*, Sportverlag Strauß, 2013.
138 Oliver Fritsch, *DDR-Dopingopfer sterben zehn bis zwölf Jahre früher*, Die Zeit, 26 March 2018.

an existence lived in the shadow of her much more famous colleagues: 'I love life but I know that I will never grow old. I am terminally ill. I am in pain. I suffer panic attacks but, in spite of that, I am optimistic. In my career I only got a fourth place at the *Spartakiade*[139] and I have never taken part in any Olympic Games or major tournament: that's why nobody knows me. My coach gave me the blue pills, but she told me they were vitamins. She cheated me. I am 44, but from a health point of view it is as if I were 80. I am gay and that's OK, but I have always wondered what my sexual life might have been without those drugs.'[140]

Many years after the end of the dreadful doping scheme, it is now reasonable to begin to consider what some doctors feared: the possible long-term consequences not just for the athletes but for their offspring too. Fortunately, it looks like most of the so-called 'Doping Grandchildren' have not inherited serious medical conditions, but there is, nonetheless, a significant number of young people who show the same side effects suffered by their parents. We have already reported Martina Gottschalt, Barbara Krause and Jutta Gottschalk's dreadful experiences with their children; here we tell Mercedes Ostrowski's story.

Mercedes (daughter of Petra, a talented canoeist who was forced to retire at 13 because of some adverse effects of the drugs on her body), has recently confessed what happened to her family: 'I have to shave in places where girls usually don't have hair. I am embarrassed to go out with my boyfriend. I think I may have trouble conceiving in the future; the doctors don't know what the long-term consequences of the doping may be. My sister Melina died aged ten because of her many congenital conditions. My mother blames herself for her

---

139 Youth national games, a really important event organised once every two years in the GDR; it was hugely popular and was attended by several thousand teenagers.

140 Oliver Fritsch, *Vergiftet von der DDR*, Die Zeit, 26 March 2018.

death, but I have told her many times that the real [person] responsible is not her.' In a declassified letter dated 4 August 1976, signed by 'Technik', we can read how Petra Ostrowski, having refused to take the 'supportive means' because they made her feel sick, had to be excluded from the sports club and also from school. This note shows once again the system's total lack of scruples towards the athletes.[141]

Petra is one of the many state-sponsored doping victims: her daughter's virilisation problems show that, at least in this particular case, the effects of those drugs could be transferred from one generation to the next.

Although women are the main victims of the doping system, there is also a significant number of sportsmen who suffered the consequences of that cruel scheme. One of them, Frank Hellmuth, a former SC Dynamo Berlin handball player, today lives with numerous pathologies, all probably correlated to the steroids he had taken years ago: 'I am just 57 but I constantly live in agony, because of the many surgical operations to my knee; I have a chronic spine condition and my joints are almost totally worn out. I survived testicular cancer but I now have prostate cancer. I know this is all because of the drugs they gave me when I was at Dynamo. I tried to discuss this problem with my former club-mates but they don't want to talk about it. One day, one of them confessed that medals are more important than the truth.'[142]

As we'll see, Hellmuth is not the only sportsman to have experienced such difficult times; his testimony hints at the fact that many others might share his conditions but, either because of pride, shame or because of the fear of losing their medals, they tend to forget and leave their controversial past alone, refusing any attempt to come to terms with their conscience.

---

141 Ibid.
142 Oliver Fritsch, *Vergiftet von der DDR*, Die Zeit, 26 March 2018.

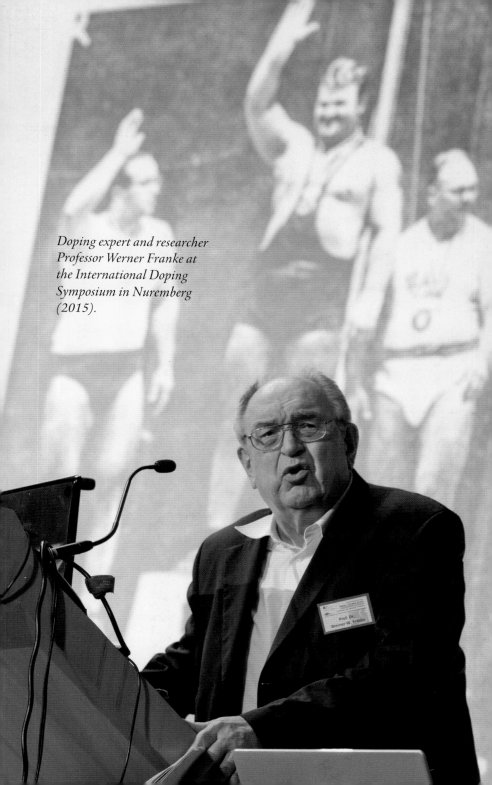

Doping expert and researcher Professor Werner Franke at the International Doping Symposium in Nuremberg (2015).

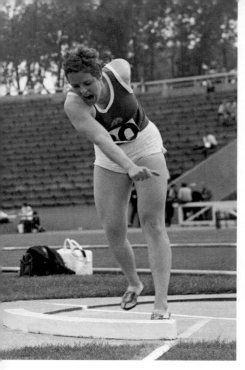

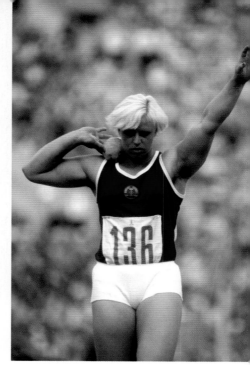

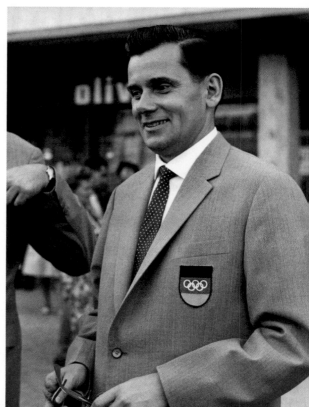

Top left: *GDR shot putter Margitta Gummel (1968).*

Top right: *GDR shot putter Ilona Slupianek at the Moscow Olympics (1980).*

Right: *Manfred Ewald, president of the central sports organisation of the GDR, the Deutscher Turn- und Sportbund (1960).*

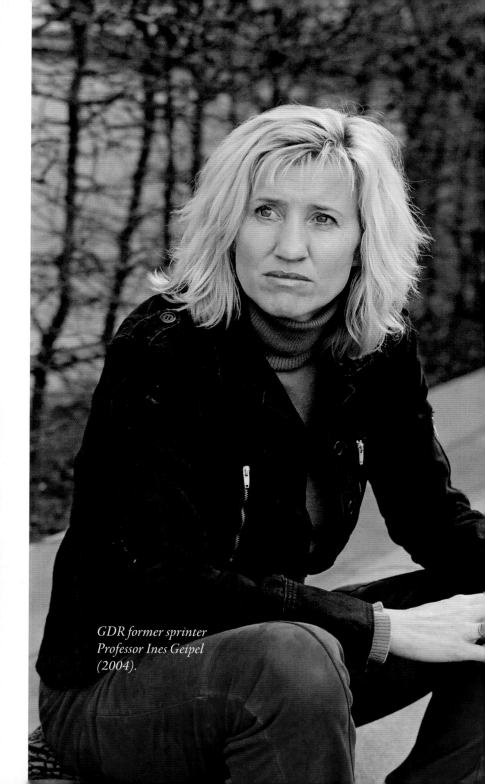

*GDR former sprinter
Professor Ines Geipel
(2004).*

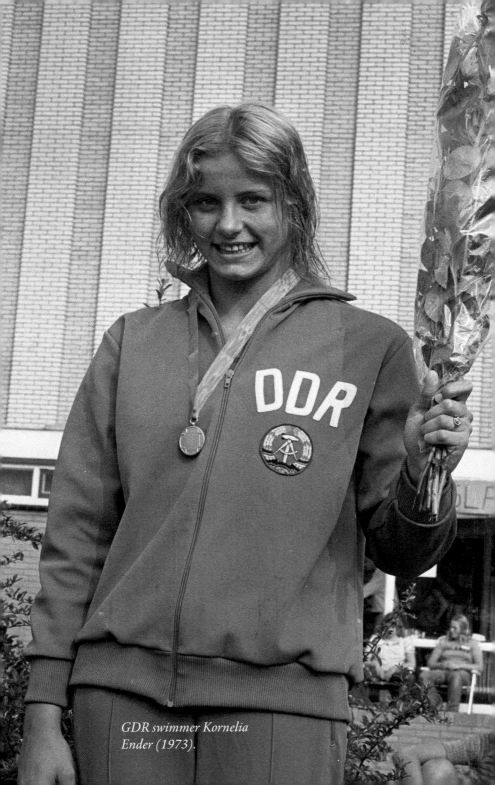

GDR swimmer Kornelia Ender (1973).

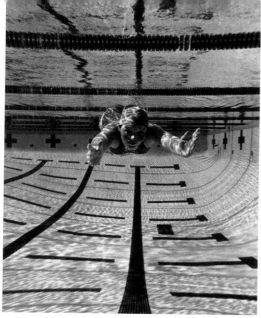

US swimmer Shirley Babashoff (1976).

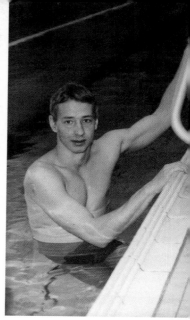

GDR swimmer Sigurd Hanke (1983).

The former GDR gymnastics athletes, Dana Boldt (left) and Susann Scheller at the HELIOS clinics in Schwerin, during a press conference on doping abuse in the GDR (2018).

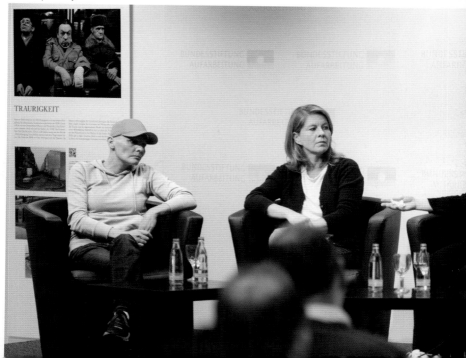

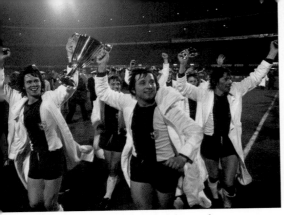

FC Magdeburg players celebrate their victory over AC Milan after the UEFA Cup Winners' Cup Final (1974).

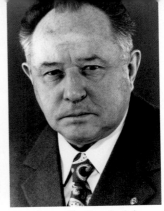

Erich Mielke, head of the East German Ministry for State Security (Stasi) *from 1957 to 1989.*

Football player Lutz Eigendorf (1980).

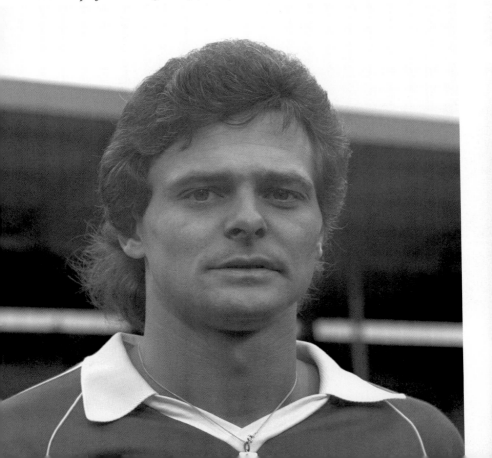

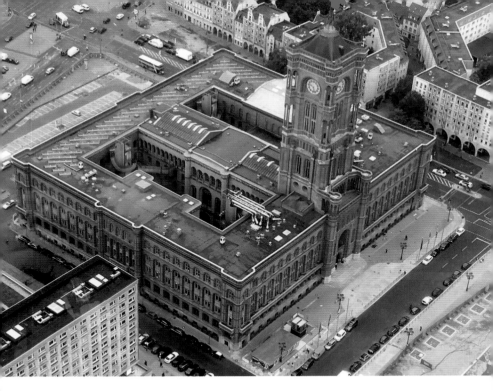

Rotes Rathaus, Berlin, headquarters of the East German Olympic Committee from 1951 to 1990 (2019).

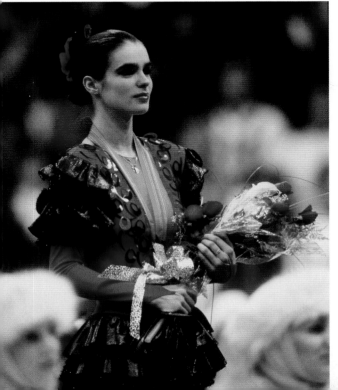

GDR skater Katarina Witt at the 1988 Olympics in Calgary.

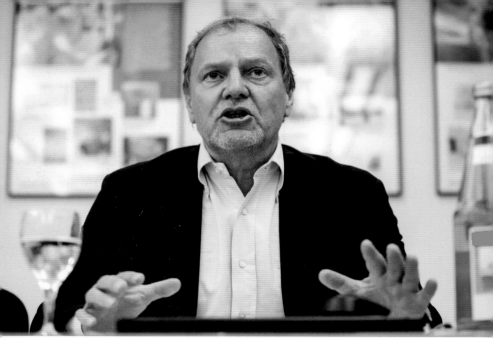

German lawyer Michael Lehner, chairman of the Doping-Opfer-Hilfe *organisation (2015)*

Michael Lehner (left), chairman of the Doping-Opfer-Hilfe *organisation, and Werner Franke, biologist and anti-doping expert, argue before the start of a press conference of the* Verein Doping-Opfer-Hilfe (DOH) *at the building entrance*

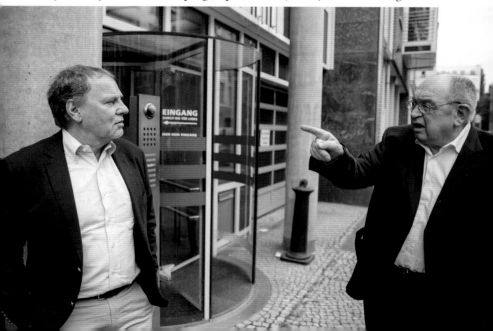

Today, Dr Sigurd Hanke, a former swimmer from Erfurt and GDR (100m and 200m breaststroke) champion, is a surgeon in a clinic near Leipzig. He started his sports career in 1977 with Marlies Grohe, a coach who was openly against doping, but a few years later things changed. 'I was 18 years old when I was shortlisted for the 1981 European Championships in Split, Yugoslavia, and became a member of the adult national team,' recalls Hanke. 'I was told by my trainer that it was time to come up with "supporting means" (UM). There was talk of vitamins and other substances, but probably not directly of Oral-Turinabol; we athletes suspected that the little light blue pills were male hormones. Was there a sense of wrongdoing on my part? I do not know anymore. Maybe there was. On the other hand, we knew that doping was taking place all over the world, otherwise there would have been no doping controls anywhere.

'Maybe I would have thought differently about it if I had reached the performance range of European or even world records – but I was far from it. For me it was about travelling, about getting out of the walled-in country, and I put up with it for that. There was no explanation whatsoever on the drugs we received. No indication of possible side effects. Not even the name of the substance. There were only rumours. We realised, by looking at our girls and at their physical and mental changes, that such hormone preparations existed. That was impressive and couldn't be overlooked. To this day I don't know what was in other remedies that were declared as vitamin powder and protein drink. Also, I don't know what was in the shots we were given.'

Young Sigurd was trapped in a sort of limbo: doping or freedom? The choice, as for many athletes, was not easy. 'It was not possible to openly reject the UM: I should have stopped competitive sports immediately, with expulsion from the KJS and back to a normal school, in which I would not have got along well because of different curricula. A dictatorship works like that, and the one in the GDR was like that too. A complete rejection was hardly possible. Therefore, whenever I could, I secretly tried not to take the pills that I was given. We weren't scared of what we thought were male hormones as boys. Why should male hormones be wrong in a young man? The only thing I had heard was that without hard training you would get fat from it. Since I didn't do any iron-hard training and didn't want to get fat, I often didn't take the pills. However, we were powerless against injections and infusions. When you are young, you are more willing to take risks. Even with drugs. Besides, how many people risked their lives at the border to get out of the country? We GDR athletes had basically no choice, if we didn't want to manoeuvre ourselves into social obscurity for the rest of our lives.'[143]

As a professional, Dr Hanke has tried to monitor and analyse his own health condition over the last 30 years: 'I have experienced various illnesses that could be directly or indirectly related to doping-forced competitive sports: Achilles tendon rupture, quadriceps tendon rupture, paroxysmal atrial fibrillation/cardiac arrhythmia, membranous glomerulonephritis, cervicolumbar syndrome, thoracic spine blockage with longitudinal ligament stiffening, lumbar spine structure loosening, sacroiliac joint arthritis, patellofemoral pain syndrome, plantar fascia contracture on both sides with metatarsalgia on both sides.'[144]

It is hard to say whether the illnesses above are all related to doping, but they certainly make an incredibly long list that together would rarely affect a single person, without a specific reason. Dr Hanke has managed, through sheer determination, to live to tell the tale; fortunately his conditions are not life-threatening. Nevertheless, pain and discomfort have surely

---

143 Correspondence with the author.
144 Correspondence with the author.

influenced his life and career from a psychological point of view: 'I have worked excessively in a self-destructive manner for many years. The professional success that came with it seemed to prove me right but, in the end, it didn't go well. After more and more physical symptoms with no somatic correlate, I sought psychological treatment. I'm fine at the moment. I can pursue my beautiful job, I can do (almost) everything I want and I enjoy it, I'm still active in sports, go swimming twice a week, go hiking.'[145]

Among the male athletes who have had a miserable life after the end of their sports career, we can't forget Gerd Bonk, surreptitiously recognised as 'the world champion of doping'. Bonk, an Olympic medallist weightlifter, is the East German sportsman who took more steroids than everyone else: the 'merit' of this record belongs to Hans-Henning Lathan, the Weightlifting Federation doctor who ignored any safety protocol and administered his athletes more drugs than normally accepted. In 1991, Latham admitted that high-performance athletes had been 'systematically administered doping agents', including drugs that had not yet been fully tested and approved.[146] According to a report by Werner Franke and Brigitte Berendonk, Bonk had taken 12,775mg of steroids during a one-year period: a huge amount. Just to have an idea of the enormity of that figure, consider that world record holder Uwe Hohn (who threw his javelin over 104m!) took 1,135mg, and Canadian sprinter Ben Johnson took 1,500mg.[147]

However, the most disturbing aspect of Bonk's career has to do with the fact that his doctors knew that by 1979 he had developed diabetes; they thought it was acceptable

---

145 Correspondence with the author.
146 *Keine Namen, aber Codezahlen*, Neues Deutschland, 6 June 1991.
147 Brian Blickenstaff, *The Rise and Fall of Gerd Bonk, the World Champion of Doping*, Bild, 10 August 2016.

to carry on with the doping programme, without telling him about his condition. Evidently, in the twisted minds of some East German officers the supreme glory of the nation outweighed the athlete's health, even when this was already compromised. Gerd Bonk found out about his diabetes only when the federation officers cancelled his participation at the Moscow Olympics, because of his high level of steroids. Soon afterwards, Bonk experienced kidney failure and ended up in a wheelchair. He couldn't even attend the *Dopingprozess* as he was too ill. He died in 2014, 'destroyed by the GDR', in his words, 'and forgotten by the united Germany'.[148] No federation officer or sportsman attended his funeral.

Psychological oppression

Life within the walls of certain East German sports clubs did not only comprise training and drugs; there was, at times, another aspect – a more sinister one – which had to do with the sadistic side of some of the officers in charge. The aforementioned Dr Harald Freyberger, psychiatrist at Helios clinic in Stralsund, suggests that almost 20 per cent of female athletes were psychologically and sexually abused.[149]

Former GDR sailor, now journalist and doping expert, Andre Keil emphasises that the quantity of verbal violence was very high in the training group he was in. Comments like 'You are too fat' or 'You look disgusting' were often used. The fact that most children were also long separated from their parents, for the training sessions, also increased their level of anxiety. Keil is convinced that those abuses led, over the years, to 'very bad illnesses at 40 or 50 years of age'.[150]

---

148 Ibid.

149 Friedhard Teuffel, *Das War Sadismus der Trainer*, Der Tagesspiegel, 3 May 2017.

150 Thomas Wheeler, *Was da zutage kommt, ist ziemlich erschütternd*, Deutschlandfunkkultur, 18 December 2016.

Rhythmic gymnast Susann Scheller tells how she and her club-mates were tormented by certain training methods: 'Sport should be fun, but to me it has always been like torture. We had to train every day, all day, until we dropped. At some point, some even tried to hurt their joints with glass bottles or injure their arms in order to have a few days off from training. When they let us go home, every two or three weeks, they would always release us late, so we had to run to the rail station and, very often, I missed my train. I had to wait four hours for the next one, alone in a dark and nearly empty station. I was only 11. My parents would wait for me for hours. Even today, I don't like travelling by train.'[151]

Like Susann Scheller, Dana Boldt is a former rhythmic gymnast who is today suffering the consequences of years of humiliating training sessions. The athlete from Frankfurt am Oder is completely bald; she lost all her hair when she was 15, probably because of the drugs she took. 'They started stuffing me with steroids when I was ten. At that age I didn't know what substances they were giving me and I didn't even wonder about them. If my parents had come to know about it, they would have gone mad. My coaches were ruthless. More than once, they took me by my neck and dragged me out of the gym because I weighed a little more than the expected standard. Training sessions were very harsh; at times we would finish at 21.30, but only because the caretaker had to close the gym to go home.'[152]

After the reunification of the two Germanys, Dana's mother went through a lot of declassified documents in order to find evidence of administration of Oral-Turinabol to her daughter, but she discovered that all papers relevant to Dana had been destroyed.

---

151 Oliver Fritsch, *Vergiftet von der DDR*, Die Zeit, 26 March 2018.
152 Peter Ahrens, *Kaputte Körper, kaputte Seelen*, Der Spiegel, 25 April 2018.

Today, Dana Boldt is 50 and suffers from depression and cardiac arrhythmia; a few years ago, encouraged by her girlfriend, she decided to tell her story at public events and conferences, where other former athletes share their problems. She has gradually started feeling better.[153] As usual, to confront our own demons is the best way to come to terms with our past, abandoning that common, weird – and wrong – sensation of feeling guilty for other people's misdemeanours.

Iris Buchholz, a talented rower who never won anything important, still retains the letters she sent from her club in East Berlin to her family in Schwerin, in 1977. In some of these you can still read all her frustration for the unreasonable behaviour of her coaches: 'Dear family, ... I should have come back home around the 19/20 November, but our coach wants us to train for the 10km distance and we have to stay at the club longer than expected. We are all upset. ... We can't even complain. It's not fair to force us to stay here until Christmas. I would kick them all.'[154]

Today, Iris Buchholz is a career woman with a good job, but she has to deal with a serious health condition caused by the drugs administered to her when she was a young girl. The former athlete found out about the *Staatsplanthema* by watching a documentary on TV. In addition to a heart condition, Iris suffers from muscle pain and depression: 'When I read my old letters, I relive the great pressure we had to endure. My coaches insulted me if I didn't go as fast as they wanted; they always told me that what I did was never enough – sport was only about winning. If we did not reach certain objectives, we were punished and we weren't allowed to go home. The *Stasi* made sure to keep us separated from our

153 Stephan Enke, *Doping in der DDR – ein Opfer erzählt*, Märkische Allgemeine, 20 February 2017.

154 Alexa Hennings, *Schaden an Leib und Seele*, Deutschlandfunkkultur, February 2020.

families as much as possible to avoid protective interference from our parents.'[155]

Buchholz's health problems started when she was a teenager; gradually, she began to lose her fitness and eventually had to stop and leave her sports club. Despite the fact that she got top grades at school, she was refused a place at university and the medical treatment she needed was denied. 'Over time, I developed a series of insecurities and became hesitant in every aspect of my life. I was proud to belong to the prestigious Dynamo Berlin club. My friends said they were envious. Now, I am sure they wouldn't be anymore. How can you be envious of someone who has a pacemaker and often stumbles to the ground for no reason?'[156]

Volleyball player Kathy Pohl also decided to share her experience of assorted pains that started at school age: 'I soon fell prey to an indescribable, intense and prolonged disease, but I didn't go to the doctor because I didn't want to be excluded from my club, Traktor Schwerin, by my coach. We all had this weird idea that the trainers might be upset if we didn't perform well, so we endured abuses of all kinds. Sometimes, instead of training in the gym, they would take us to an outdoor military training camp; we used this to test defence schemes: we had to practise defending against spikes by diving into pebbles and mud. At the end of the training session, our legs were bruised all over. Nobody dared to protest.'[157]

Kathy, who lives with a few neurological disabilities, learned from her family doctor that she had taken steroids for years, when she visited him to get a statement of disability. The doctor, once he learned Kathy played for Traktor Schwerin, revealed she was certainly given steroids. 'I denied it. I was sure I didn't take anything but the doctor told me

---

155 Ibid.
156 Ibid.
157 Ibid.

he had seen many former athletes from my club, all showing the same illnesses, at the Rostock Hospital, and they had all taken steroids.' Kathy Pohl was clearly shocked; she had gone to see her doctor for a routine visit and she came out with a revelation which turned her life upside down.[158] Iris Buchholz and Kathy Pohl today live in Schwerin, capital city of Mecklenburg-Vorpommern (a state in north Germany), along the Baltic Sea coast. Here, the local government has taken the decision to provide concrete help to the victims of state doping. The first port of call is a counselling centre managed by Dr Daniela Richter: we will discuss this scheme in detail in the final chapter.

Former gymnast Esther Nicklas still struggles to talk about an episode she witnessed as a young girl, 30 years ago: 'We were training in the gym, when at a certain moment we heard a piercing scream. At first, we did not understand where it came from, then we saw a team-mate in pain under the asymmetrical parallels; she must have been hurt very much, but the first thing our coach did was to mute her mouth. The more she squirmed, the more he prevented her from moving and crying. How could he do it? How could someone restrain a girl in pain? That scene still haunts me.'[159] Obviously, the other girls couldn't be distracted by such unpleasant accidents and they had to keep focusing on their routines, coldly and efficiently.

Nicklas, together with former team-mates Dörte Thümmler, Manuela Renk and Susann Scheller, also reports a disturbing situation going on at the club: athletes who were good enough to pursue a world-level career would find it very difficult to leave the institution. Even despite an assortment of joint and muscular pains, girls couldn't quit when they wished; the sports club would, in fact, put their families under

---

158 Ibid.

159 Interview in the documentary 'Der Kraftakt': Folgen des DDR-Leistungssport-systems, by Andre Keil and Benjamin Unger, NDR, 2018.

great pressure to convince their children to carry on with their sports activities and achieve excellent results. Although there is no reason to doubt this account, other former athletes have also said that it wasn't so difficult for them to leave their club, when the time came; as usual, in East Germany, rules and regulations, and their implementation, depended on circumstances, places and the nature of the people involved.

Regarding the difficulties in leaving the sports clubs, for Gabriele Fähnrich the most exciting aspect of her experience at the Olympics in Seoul in 1988 was not the bronze medal she won, but the fact that those Games marked her last appearance in a sports event. The GDR coaches were finally happy with her performances and her career – Fähnrich had also won the World Championship – and they decided to release her from her duties and keep the promise they made a few years earlier, giving her the chance to attend a beautician's course in the most renowned school in East Berlin. However, getting to that moment of freedom had not been easy, as the gymnast recalls: 'The last few years at Dynamo had been gruelling. I often had pain in my knees, but instead of letting me rest, they would inject me with some "miracle" drug that helped me to heal quickly, but in the long term it caused me even more pain. Years later, after reading a newspaper article, I realised that they were pumping me with steroids. At some point, during the peak of my sports career, I had made the decision to give up gymnastics; I was immediately summoned to a meeting with the big-wigs at Dynamo, who gave me a two-hour lecture on the consequences I would have to pay if I had left – I would be dishonourably discharged and my parents would lose their apartment and car. Eventually, I was forced to stay. When I did my last competition in Seoul, I was very happy.'[160]

---

160 Beatrice Zajda, *Für Medaillen die Gesundheit ruiniert*, Deutschlandfunkkultur, October 2019.

One of the most dreaded aspects in sports institutions was nutrition. As Susann Scheller recalls, girls had to be exactly the weight their coaches wanted: they sometimes made them fast, while on other occasions they stuffed them with food: 'One day, they tested us with apple pies on a table. Those of us who dared to eat a slice were forced into endless runs. Some girls became anorexic.'[161]

Hard training, blackmail, steroids and odd diets were a bad enough combination for those girls and it's no wonder that many of them today suffer from various diseases and have neurological conditions. The environment where Susann, Kathy, Gabriele, Esther and countless others had to live and grow up was certainly not suitable for adults, let alone for children.

Unfortunately, as anticipated above, for Susann Scheller there was one more dark aspect to consider: 'The most traumatic place was Zinnowitz, a special training camp on Usedom, an island in the Baltic Sea. When we ran on the beach, our coach would sometimes order us to get in the water for a swimming session. We had to undress completely. After years, I learned that one of the doctors was spying on us from afar, hidden behind the dunes. In the evening, the same doctor invited us one by one to his room. One day, he asked me to undress. I remained in my underwear. I don't remember exactly what happened next. Some say that it was sexual abuse. Frankly, I don't know what to say. I only know that that hazy memory continues to haunt me.'[162]

Recently, Scheller formed a WhatsApp group with her former team-mates to share their experiences and try to pursue possible complaints, even after such a long time, against their abusers.

---

161 Oliver Fritsch, *Vergiftet von der DDR*, Die Zeit, 26 March 2018.
162 Ibid.

Incredibly, the psychological harassment of athletes continued, in some cases, even after the fall of the Berlin Wall. Despite the ongoing restructuring and reshaping of various sports clubs in 1990, there was one, SC Magdeburg, which managed (thanks to some influential characters connected with local politicians) to keep its athletes under control and survive for a couple more years after '*Die Wende*'. At the 1989 European Swimming Championships, in Bonn, some top athletes, including Anke Möhring (three gold medals) and Kathleen Nord (one gold and one bronze), came from the Saxony club. After that event, both being aged 18, the two girls wanted to abandon the club and continue with their academic studies, but the political and psychological pressures from their coaches and managers were such that Anke and Kathleen had to accept an unconscionable contract: they had to keep competing for the club with the vague promise of a university scholarship and a salary of 400 marks. When the SC Magdeburg officials failed to keep their side of the deal, Anke Möhring revealed the club's vexatious actions to the local press.

With a final blow, the club executives, no longer able to entrust their athletes to the 'loving care' of the *Stasi*, decided to resort to gossip of the lowest order: they managed to convince the local press to publish slanderous articles mentioning that Möhring had become a 'bartender' in a well-known red-light nightclub.

A disgusting rumour, obviously, but in the end it fell on deaf ears because the bar in question had already been closed for some time. Fortunately, just a few years later, the diligent East German elite would finally lose the ability to threaten and harass people. The fact that Anke and Kathleen succeeded in leaving their club without trouble didn't save them from one final insult: in 1992, the scholarships 'promised' by the Magdeburg's bosses were in fact cancelled by the united Germany.

Football, doping and the *Stasi*

Although the most important successes for East Germany often came from athletics and swimming, the most popular sport was football and doping was also present in this sport, but the Federation's key directive was very specific about it: pharmaceutical substances (generally steroids and amphetamines) should only be used for matches involving the national team and the clubs taking part in European (UEFA) competitions. Given that football's degree of creativity could not be enhanced by pharmaceutical supports, attempts were made to limit their use.[163] In addition, the football system was so complex and extensive, with so many clubs, players and coaches, that it would have been very difficult to keep doses under control and to avoid news leaks about illegal practices. In 1966, in fact, following a match against Hungary, the East German players were beset by sudden drowsiness, raising doubts and suspicions among journalists and observers.[164] *Stasi* documents show a list of matches in which East German players took 'supporting substances'. For example, psychostimulants such as oxytocin, mesocarb and aponeuron were certainly used for the national team's matches against Poland and Switzerland (both in 1983), and that of Dynamo Dresden against Partizan Belgrade (European Cup, 1979), and Dynamo Berlin against Werder Bremen (European Cup, 1988). Despite the aforementioned ban on drugs for league matches, several players from Dynamo Berlin, Lokomotiv Leipzig, Dynamo Dresden and Magdeburg were found to have positive urine tests at the Keischa laboratory, run by the well-known Dr Manfred Höppner.[165] The *Deutscher Fußball Verband* executives were very angry about that 'unauthorised'

---

163 Mike Dennis and Jonathan Grix, *Sport Under Communism – Behind the East German Miracle*, Palgrave Macmillan, 2012.

164 Mike Dennis, *Doping in East German Football since the 1960s*, published on Balticworlds.com, 19 June 2012.

165 Ibid.

practice and threatened some players with disqualification. Years later, researcher Giselher Spitzer discovered that football players took doping unknowingly.[166] Two of them, Falko Götz and Dirk Schlegel, had managed to escape to West Germany, and Höppner's fear was that they could reveal the secrets of certain 'chemical practices' to their new team-mates or, worse, to the foreign press. The news of that defection was so bad that Höppner and his direct *Stasi* controller preferred not to let the irascible Manfred Ewald know about it. In any case, the unauthorised use of doping had triggered an alarm among the managers of the DTSB, prompting more restrictive measures and surprise checks.[167] In short, doping was allowed, but in moderation and without breaking the rules. It seems incredible how the country that had instigated the use of doping as a 'state religion' took action to fight it; but these things happened in the variegated and contradictory world of the GDR.

Apart from some important successes, such as winning the gold medal at the Montréal Olympics and Magdeburg's victory in the Cup Winners' Cup (beating Italian giants AC Milan in the final in 1974), East Germany's footballers didn't achieve the same level of results as the swimming or athletics clubs; the victory of the Saxony side must in fact be considered unique in the context of European club tournaments. The architect of that sensational win was Heinz Krügel, considered at the time one of the best managers in Europe, to the point that the Italian club Juventus offered him a four-million-mark contract, with a bonus if he managed to persuade Magdeburg forward Martin Hoffmann to move to Turin as well. Moving to Italy would have been really complicated for an East German player; Krügel refused Juventus's tempting offer anyway, but the mere fact that he had considered that

---

166 https://www.faz.net/aktuell/sport/doping-historiker-ddr-dopte-ganze-fussball-mannschaften-1146759.html

167 Mike Dennis, *Doping in East German Football since the 1960s*, published on Balticworlds.com, 19 June 2012.

opportunity cast him in a bad light in the eyes of the top executives of East German football.

Final proof of Krügel's loyalty to true sporting values and morals came during a 1974 European Cup match against Bayern Munich. *Stasi* agents installed bugs inside the Bavarian players' dressing room, and asked Krügel to use them to pick up the tactics of their coach, Udo Lattek. But the Magdeburg coach refused to eavesdrop on his opponents, thus choosing to send his team on to the pitch without using any confidential information. The *Stasi* was not happy with that insubordination and asked the Magdeburg chairman to fire Krügel. However, removing such a popular and successful character, the idol of many fans, was not easy, even in East Germany. The patient men of the *Ministerium* had to wait for two years before getting rid of him, taking advantage of a series of negative results. From that moment on, Krügel fell out of favour and never worked again in the *Oberliga*, the East German 'Premier League'. After the reunification of the two Germanys, and many years of alienation, the old coach was fully rehabilitated by the DFB, the German Football Association. Heinz Krügel was reinstated to the Magdeburg management staff, where he remained until his death in 2008. The following year, the Saxony municipality decided to dedicate the square in front of the stadium to him, and erect a striking bronze statue representing the manager holding the Cup Winners' Cup.

At national level, apart from the 'moderate' use of drugs, there were always great political manoeuvres to influence the results of this or that club. It is known that Erich Mielke, the very powerful head of the Ministry of Security with an obscure past (and responsible, among other things, for the murder of two policemen at Bülowplatz in 1931),[168] was a

---

168 Wolfgang Zank, *Der Mann, der alle liebte*, Die Zeit, 14 November 2007.

great football fan, and he made good use of his position to help his club, Dynamo Berlin, triumph in the *Oberliga*. The referees were often 'encouraged' to make decisions in favour of Mielke's team (e.g. giving non-existent penalties) and against their opponents (e.g. by showing yellow and red cards when the opportunity arose). Bernd Heynemann, a former East German referee in the 1980s, clarified candidly that 'if Dynamo lost a match, immediately afterwards the referee would be called by Mielke and be reminded that such a thing should never happen again'.[169] Former Dynamo Berlin striker Falko Götz also confessed that the referees always treated his team favourably due to the enormous pressure from the Ministry of Security. Under Mielke's watchful eye, Dynamo succeeded in the incredible feat of winning ten championships in a row!

The *Stasi* boss was very protective of his players and, when they had to go abroad for European competitions, they often travelled in his personal jet. The players were being watched all the time by intelligence agents – Mielke wanted to avoid, at all costs, his stars deciding to take advantage of the trips to defect to West Germany or some other European country.

The implementation of tight controls was due to the fact that some players had already fled over the Wall. One of them, Lutz Eigendorf, managed to sneak away from the rest of his team after playing a friendly match with Kaiserslautern in West Germany on 19 March 1979. Eigendorf, who had left his wife Gabriele and his daughter Sandy in Berlin, joined the Rhineland club and tried to help the rest of his family defect as well.

Lutz did not have an easy time in the West: FIFA fined him for leaving his club without permission and, at the request of Dynamo, he was also disqualified for one year. In

---

169 David Crossland, *Dynamo Berlin: The soccer club 'owned' by the Stasi*, CNN, 8 November 2019.

Kaiserslautern, Lutz bumped into fellow GDR countrymen who had managed to escape from the East years earlier in search of a new life, such as former boxer Karl-Heinz Felgner, a fellow national he met by chance in a pub. Felgner helped him to adapt to the new social context.[170] After the year's suspension, Lutz Eigendorf started playing in the first team but, within a few years, a series of injuries consigned him to a mediocre career. He moved to Eintracht Braunschweig and on the evening of 5 March 1983, after witnessing the defeat of his team from the bench, Lutz crashed his Alfa Romeo into a tree. The footballer died two days later from serious injuries sustained in the road accident.

As documents in the *Stasi* archives reveal, Erich Mielke had taken Eigendorf's desertion very badly and had unleashed about 50 secret agents to locate him. One of these was Karl-Heinz Felgner, the old boxer Lutz met 'by chance' in a pub. In 2009, Felgner confessed to a judge that he was actually ordered to approach and assassinate Eigendorf, but he eventually refused to execute the killing.[171]

A documentary produced by journalist Heribert Schwan, and broadcast by the German network ARD, proposes the hypothesis that Eigendorf was actually murdered by the *Stasi* for betraying his country, through the simulation of a road accident.[172] Declassified documents, albeit fragmentary and incomplete, suggest that the Berlin footballer may have been drugged before being positioned by someone behind the wheel of his car. There is also mention of a truck that was supposed to crash into a bend. The autopsy had revealed a particularly high alcohol level, but the testimonies of some friends with

---

170 Alessandro Mastroluca, *La valigia dello sport. La storia del Novecento riletta attraverso imprese e personaggi sportivi indimenticabili*, Effepi Libri, 2012.

171 Uli Hesse-Lichtenberger, *The curious case of Lutz Eigendorf, Part 2*, ESPN FC, 2 March 2010.

172 Ibid.

whom he had spent the evening at the pub said Eigendorf had only had a couple of beers. Besides, the road he was on wasn't his usual route home. In some *Stasi* documents, we can see that two agents assigned to follow Eigendorf received 500 francs each as an unspecified payment. In short, Schwan's documentary highlights the possibility of a cover-up, with an assortment of errors and omissions during the inquiry; the journalist proposes, 30 years after Eigendorf's death, the reopening of the investigation.[173]

Regardless of Schwan's conclusions, the documents once again demonstrate the climate of control, paranoia and suspicion that permeated the air in East Germany. Going against a guy like Mielke was dangerous enough; it would not be entirely unexpected if, one day, it is confirmed that Eigendorf's car accident was one of the many personal vendettas carried out by the notorious statesman.

In March 1986, Dynamo Dresden, a club from the capital city of Saxony, were experiencing one of the best moments in their history, having qualified for the quarter-finals of the UEFA Cup Winners' Cup. They had to face Bayer Uerdingen, a club from Krefeld, West Germany. The epilogue of the double confrontation has gone down in the history of European football as one of the most incredible and controversial. After winning the first leg at home 2-0, two weeks later, Dynamo found themselves 3-1 up at half-time in the second leg, at Krefeld. With the semi-final practically in their pockets, Dynamo managed the absurd 'feat' of conceding six goals in 30 minutes and therefore getting eliminated from the competition, against all odds. The post-game hours spent in the hotel were hectic; Dynamo striker Frank Lippmann took the opportunity to escape from police surveillance and managed to reach Nuremberg, where he had some relatives.

---

173 Alessandro Mastroluca, *La valigia dello sport. La storia del Novecento riletta attraverso imprese e personaggi sportivi indimenticabili*, Effepi Libri, 2012.

Soon after, the West German club 1.FC Nuremberg offered him a one-year contract.

Lippmann, who had abandoned his wife and child, was deeply vilified at home and declared a traitor, but unlike in the case of Eigendorf, the *Stasi* decided, this time, to adopt a softer approach. As soon as they tracked down the renegade footballer, they offered him a sort of amnesty if he would agree to spy on Nuremberg players on behalf of the GDR. Lippmann not only refused but, through some friends, he managed to organise the escape of his wife and son via Hungary and Austria. The East German agents would find it difficult to approach the player again. A document found in the *Stasi* archives contained an officer's comment regarding the Lippmann case, which is mercilessly revealing: '… certain traitors should be eliminated as soon as possible through a false road accident'.[174]

Doug Gilbert's last run

Yes, you are right: the name 'Doug Gilbert' doesn't sound exactly German. In addition, in this instance the word 'run' doesn't even refer to an Olympic sports event. Doug Gilbert is, in fact, a Canadian journalist. On 9 July 1979, at about 7.30pm, he had just finished writing his article for the *Edmonton Sun,* an account of the ninth day of the Pan-American Games in San Juan, Puerto Rico. He wanted to make it special and it took a little longer than expected. The USA, as usual, were winning the most medals, but Canada were doing well behind them and Cuba; perhaps, the Canucks would be able to finish third in the medals table. An intense heat, reinforced by the dazzling sunlight that penetrated low through the windows of the smoky Holiday Inn press room, was not abated at all by the few rusty fans scattered around

---

174 MDR Zeitreise, *DDR-Fußballer – Flucht als 'Verrat'*, 1 November 2010.

the hall. The organisers had promised air conditioners. Never mind! They would be ready for next time, maybe. Of course, it would be a long time before San Juan could host such an important sports event again. However, the Puerto Rican capital had done an excellent job; the organisation lived up to an event that hosts athletes from all over the American continent, from Canada to Argentina. Doug loved his job and he was having fun.

But the day wasn't over yet. There were some important races to watch in the evening. Doug had to rush to the Sixto Escobar stadium to see the climax of the women's pentathlon event. He could not miss it: a compatriot, Diane Jones-Konihowski, was in the lead and hoped to grab the gold medal. Diane was also a friend. Unfortunately, the last bus to the stadium had already left, but Doug, who had been a decent athlete in his youth, decided to run to the sports complex – it would only take 15 minutes. No big deal. Besides, the air was now a little cooler and the avenue leading to the stadium was in the shade.

He began his first 100m at a brisk but steady pace.

Then, darkness.

Doug was suddenly run over by a Volkswagen Beetle and ended up on the dusty tarmac. The rescuers quickly understood that his condition was quite serious and he was rushed to the Presbyterian Hospital but, after two hours of agony, he died, just as the Canadian national anthem reverberated at the Sixto Escobar to celebrate the victory of his friend, Diane.

A freak accident had therefore tragically put an end to the earthly existence of Doug Gilbert, a familiar face of Canadian journalism, author of important reports on the world of sport; winner of numerous awards, such as the Sportswriter of the Year, in 1977, and the prestigious National Newspaper Award (a sort of Canadian Pulitzer Prize), in 1978. Gilbert's determination and competence had allowed him to become the only reporter from the entire Western world to have access to the East German sports facilities three times, and to interview its managers and athletes. The fruits of about three years of methodical work would be published in two posthumous works: the book *The Miracle Machine* and a documentary produced and directed by Paula S. Aspell, titled *Race for Gold*. Doug Gilbert's book, a detailed account of the GDR's sports system, is the centre around which mysterious events and disturbing characters revolve.

Gilbert's killer, a certain Richard Drousse, spent the night at the San Juan police station, but he was released the next day, without formal charges. Drousse declared that he suddenly found Gilbert in front of his Volkswagen and that he could not do anything to avoid him. The journalist's death was filed as an accident; there were no witnesses, and Drousse was cleared of any responsibility. Case closed.

Years later, a mysterious person contacted some of Doug's close relatives, revealing that the reporter's death wasn't an accident and that the journalist was actually killed by the Cuban secret police, carrying out orders from the *Stasi*.

Evidence? None.

However, that weird encounter alarmed the Gilbert family. Investigative journalists Alan Freeman and Karin Helmstaedt, who worked for the Canadian newspaper the *Globe and Mail*, tried to find out more. They discovered that Gilbert, during the last days of his life, was working on the final draft of his book, *The Miracle Machine*, and that he had announced shock revelations about the 'pharmaceutical habits' of the East German sports executives. Is it possible that the Canadian reporter had learned about the GDR state-sponsored doping programme and intended to reveal it in his book? If so, is it possible that the *Stasi* had discovered his intentions and had decided to silence him with the usual planned car accident?[175]

---

175 Alan Freeman and Karin Helmstaedt, *The writer, the steroids and the Stasi*, The Globe and Mail, 12 February 2000 and updated with new material on 25 March 2018.

Six months after the journalist's death, *The Miracle Machine* was edited by his publishers, Coward, McCann & Geoghegan, and put on sale, but there was no trace in it of the much-heralded exclusive revelation. I have read Gilbert's book; my personal impression is that, however well-written and finely researched and argued, in places it looks like a sort of celebration of the glorious East German sports system, to the point that the publication, in many of its parts, could be mistaken for an official editorial product of the GDR. The book's introduction says: 'How have they done it? ... The answer, sad to say for those who would like to see a devious Communist plot behind every gold medal, and a series of Frankenstanian experiments and secret drugs behind every world record, is neither sensational nor miraculous. It is simply the result of some very thorough planning by a government that (1) gives sport a higher priority than it is given anywhere else in the world; (2) seriously promotes the unified development of both mass sport for the total population and elite sport for the international-level performer; (3) has processed more than 8,000 professional coaches through the Leipzig Institute ...; (4) has certified more than 200,000 volunteer coaches ... and (5) has placed the country's medical research system at the disposal of Sport. This is the system, so envied by the West.'[176]

Indeed, reading the book, it seems that the scoop that the journalist had announced was somehow altered or removed altogether (if it ever existed) during the review process, before going to print. Is this assumption good enough to support the idea of a conspiracy? Alan Freeman and Karin Helmstaedt considered the possibility of foul play and went to Germany to examine the *Stasi* files. They found out that Doug Gilbert had won the trust of the GDR authorities, who allowed him to

---

176 Doug Gilbert, *The Miracle Machine*, Coward, McCann & Geoghegan, New York, 1980.

enter their sports facilities and ask questions. However, Doug was also carefully spied on by a series of agents who reported that the Canadian journalist was in effect a trustworthy person. As we have seen, in the early 1970s, East Germany was trying to establish itself on the world sports scene and the idea that an esteemed and well-known Western journalist, adequately controlled, could write articles in their favour was considered a useful operation of international public relations. The Western nations would read about the successful application of the socialist system and the ability of its managers and coaches, at practically no cost for the East Germans.

At some point, the *Stasi* must have found out what Gilbert intended to write in his book; after the journalist met with a certain Dr Wuschech, the organisation suspected he came to know something about the doping programme. The *Stasi* tried to dissuade Gilbert from writing about that topic in his book through one of their informers, Wolfgang Gitter, a *Neues Deutschland* sports reporter. It appears that Doug didn't have any intention of modifying his book.[177]

Unfortunately, we don't know anything about the parts the *Stasi* wanted to modify, or if Doug actually changed them in the end. What we know is that, after Gilbert's death, his publishers decided to publish his book, after consulting with the GDR authorities.

The story is certainly intriguing, but unfortunately it ends with an unresolved cliffhanger. The hypothesis that Doug Gilbert was aware of the East German doping system and that he was eliminated by the *Stasi* for refusing to remove that information from his book is certainly disturbing. Aside from the curiosity of the two investigative reporters, Freeman and Helmstaedt, and of course the Gilbert family, no authority has ever felt it necessary to reopen the case. Officially, the

---

177 Alan Freeman and Karin Helmstaedt, *The writer, the steroids and the Stasi*, The Globe and Mail, 12 February 2000 and updated with new material on 25 March 2018.

circumstances that led to Doug Gilbert's death are that of a car accident, due to an unlucky moment of distraction: just an unfortunate fate, yet an incredible coincidence ominously favourable to the East German authorities.

Coaches in the mirror

As pointed out in previous chapters, the ultimate responsibility for supplying pharmaceutical aids, in the years of state-sponsored doping, was with the coaches. These were figures of the utmost importance: in daily contact with the athletes, they had to earn the young people's respect and trust. Their main burden was the constant betrayal of the very children they had to take care of, passing off the nefarious 'supporting substances' as simple vitamins. Many coaches live with remorse for what they did and they rarely wish to evoke their past. Elke Stange-Schrempf, rhythmic gymnastics coach, is one of the very few trainers who has decided to recall the events of that period. Elke does not find it difficult to expose her regret for the wicked choices she made in the 1980s: 'I have a recurring nightmare: I'm still a coach, I go to my girls lined up on the mat, and I go to shake their hand, but they refuse it. ... When I was operating in Leipzig, I was a good coach. I forged champions, but I was also too ambitious. I suspected that doctors and other coaches might be providing drugs to the girls, but I never did anything to investigate or stop them. I was just thinking about myself and my career. I should have protected them. They were so young. I never gave them anything, no pills, no syringes. Never. But I feel equally responsible.'[178]

Schrempf has recently had the chance to meet gymnast Susann Scheller. The meeting was particularly moving. Scheller talked for hours with her former coach – together they tried to tame their demons forever. 'I'm really happy

---

178 Oliver Frisch, *Vergiftet von der DDR*, Die Zeit, 26 March 2018.

that Susann decided to speak to me; many probably would have sent me a picture of them with a middle finger on display. I apologised to her and she accepted it. I would like to ask forgiveness from the other girls and reveal to them the question that will torment me until the end of my days: "Why didn't I do anything?"'[179]

From some of the testimonies reported in this book, it appears clear that not all the GDR doctors and coaches had blindly colluded with the system. We are sure that under 'normal' conditions many of them would never have distributed drugs to children; they too, albeit in different ways, were victims of the doping system. Unlike the athletes, however, they will forever be forced to deal with their own consciences.

In the variegated kaleidoscope of blameworthy characters that gravitated around the dark years of East German sport, there are some who, instead, have a clear conscience and can look in the mirror with pride, having made the morally right choice when political conditions and social situations did not easily allow it.

Among the coaches who really tried hard to shield their athletes from doping, we would like to mention Marlies Grohe, a swimming trainer who was active during the 1960s and 70s at SC Turbine Erfurt, a small civil club with weak links to the central government, a feature that kept it, for a while, away from the state-sponsored doping plan. In her youth, Grohe was a successful breaststroke swimmer, setting 100m and 200m GDR records. As a trainer, her most important achievement was discovering and managing Roland Matthes, who, under her wing, became the most successful backstroke swimmer of all time. Matthes's wins were achieved when the *Staatsplanthema* wasn't fully implemented; besides, his coach, Grohe, was famous for her negative view on doping.

---

179 Ibid.

Matthes is indeed considered by many to be one of the few 'true' champions of the GDR.

However, with time, the 'magic blue pills' reached the small Thuringian city, but Marlies Grohe stood her ground against the East German sports officials.[180] She did everything she could to protect her young athletes from the lure of doping. Sigurd Hanke was one of her boys and passionately describes her approach: 'When I started competitive sports in 1977, I was already 14 years old. I didn't go the usual route of TZ and KJS admission as a primary school child. That had to do with the idea of a "special path", which my first trainer, Marlies Grohe, implemented; she had put together a "special training group" with older children/adolescents, some of whom then switched to KJS in 1977, like me. She used to say that children do not have to start swimming so young (primary school age). Marlies Grohe was a very special pedagogue; she was empathic and warm-hearted but strict at the same time. She managed us with wisdom and competence. We loved her for being straightforward, too. She was upright in every sense. To me, she was the most important person of trust during my career as a sportsman and as a teenager as well. The details and reasons why she quit her engagement as a trainer never became clear to me. We had our presumptions, and there were some rumours, but I do not know for sure.'[181]

Grohe's views obviously went against the strategies of the existing child-recruitment system and the administration of 'supportive means'; her subversive belief wouldn't go unnoticed. In 1981, the GDR sports executives finally caught up with her. After Matthes's retirement, the club wasn't as successful as before; something had to be done to improve results. When

---

180 Karin Helmstaedt, *Swimming against the current*, The Whig-Standard, 5 May 2007.

181 Correspondence with the author.

Grohe refused to administer doping to her swimmers, she had to leave her position at the club. Regrettably, she died young, soon after the fall of the Berlin Wall, and didn't have the chance to speak about the circumstances surrounding her dismissal.

Henrich Misersky taught sports at the University of Ilmenau in the early 80s, when he was asked to revive the fortunes of SC Motor Zella-Mehlis, a women's cross-country ski club, with which his daughter Antje also raced. Around the second half of the 80s, before starting his annual training programme on the snow-covered slopes of the Thuringian Forest, Misersky was summoned to a meeting with the various leaders of the national ski team. 'We were all gathered in an anonymous hall. Here, Kurt Hinze [head of the ski coaches] and his assistant told us in no uncertain terms that from then on, athletes should take Oral-Turinabol,' recalls Misersky, 'as it had just been established for canoeists.

Until then, skiers had remained immune to doping, but that was about to change. Even my daughter was going to be pumped with steroids. To me it was unacceptable. Disgusted, I confessed to some colleagues that I would never give my athletes any "supportive means". A few spies reported my outburst.

'At first, they tried to convince me with tempting promises of promotions, but I refused. Kurt Hinze himself was forced to intervene. In a particularly fiery encounter, he literally said to me: "People like you are politically unreliable and should go away." Just six weeks after that meeting, I was fired. Before leaving, however, I informed my athletes of the nefarious plans that the leaders of the Federation had in store for them.

'I also thoroughly informed them about the consequences steroids have on the female body – I was able to get that information from my mother-in-law, a doctor. I don't know what happened to the girls, but I know for a fact that my daughter Antje went to tell the club boss that she would never compete with the help of chemistry. She was expelled from the ski team and had to train alone.'[182]

In 1985, Antje had won the bronze medal in the 4x5km relay at the Nordic World Ski Championships in Seefeld.[183] Even the documents found by Werner Franke and Brigitte Berendonk attest that that victory was clean. Despite the good results, Antje was never again called up by the GDR for international competitions.

With the unification of the two Germanys, she re-joined the national team in the speciality of biathlon, winning a gold medal and two silver medals at the Albertville Olympics, in 1992. Here, during a live broadcast, Antje's father, Henrich, had an altercation with Helmuth Weinbuch, sporting director of the German Ski Federation; he accused him of including in his team many former East German doctors and coaches who were notorious promoters of doping practices. Following that TV appearance, the Misersky family were the subject of anonymous letters containing death threats, fortunately without real intentions. For their efforts against doping, both Henrich and Antje were awarded the 'Heidi Krieger Medal', an honour given by the Doping-Opfer-Hilfe association, which we will discuss extensively in the final chapter.

Sifting through the thousands of secret *Stasi* documents, Werner Franke finds an old handwritten letter, dated 1963. The letter was sent by Johanna Sperling, a rowing coach, to her athletes at the SC DHfK Leipzig club. The message is a heartfelt appeal to female canoeists to resist the temptation to take doping substances: 'I seriously ask you not to ingest pills that can increase your performance, even if they tell you that they are perfectly harmless. Even if they tell you that you are

---

182 Henrich Misersky, *Wir haben nicht mitgemacht*, Tagesspiegel, 19 July 2009.
183 With Manuela Drescher, Gaby Nestler and Ute Noack.

the only one who does not take them, you must resist. Just focus on your races and your health. Yes, at the beginning you might see improvements, but trust me: they are not good at all.'[184]

The letter, also found by one of Sperling's former athletes, 45 years later, is delivered to Jens Weinreich, a journalist with *Der Spiegel*, who manages to track down the coach. Sperling reveals that in the 60s, before the introduction of steroids, there were attempts to introduce psychotropic substances in sports: 'Many of my colleagues were more intent on attending pharmaceutical conferences than sports seminars. Some doctors had told me about the possible side effects of those drugs. I refused to give them to my girls. I was marginalised and then relegated to junior teams. Despite those errors, however, I do not feel I can totally condemn the GDR. After all, I was a true socialist and my country had given me everything. As a young canoeist I had won a bronze medal at the European Championships, in 1957, then I graduated as a physical education teacher. But winning with doping? I was not convinced. If you can't win without the help of drugs, how can you say you've won honestly?'[185] Johanna Sperling's question has an obvious moral connotation; but in East Germany, and more broadly in the world of sports, as we have seen, there is very little room for such consideration.

The various testimonies we have seen show that the synthetic medals forged in the pharmaceutical laboratories of Jenapharm have more than two sides. On each side is reflected the determination of a country to impose itself on the international scene, the ambition of an athlete to surf the low wave of an ephemeral success, the reluctance of a teenager to following a dreadful diet, the professional exclusion of an

---

184 Jens Weinreich, '*Ich bitte euch, kein Mittelchen zu schlucken*', Der Spiegel, 18 August 2009.

185 Ibid.

honest coach, or the careerism of obscure bureaucrats, whose dream is to obtain social privileges unimaginable for many fellow citizens, such as a 70m² apartment near Alexander Platz, eating the rare oranges and bananas, or owning a snappy Trabant (the terrifying car with a two-stroke engine, popularly defined as a 'cardboard car'). Some tried to shine their own light and free themselves from the repressive embrace of the doping system but, as we have seen, they were left in the dark. However, time has proven that their inner light was powerful and, after many years of oblivion, in the end, prevailed. The exasperation of getting excellent results at all costs shines, instead, like black light that refracts inside the bodies of young athletes, used and sacrificed on the altar of a distorted ideology, but always following the dictates of 'brotherhood and civil coexistence' of socialism. As Manfred Ewald himself said: 'We don't want to hurt our athletes at all, but we have to take some risks.'[186]

---

186 K. Marxen, G. Werle, *Strafjustiz und DDR-Unrecht. Dokumentation. Band 7: Gefangenenmisshandlung, Doping und sostiges DDR-Unrecht*, De Gruyter Recht, 2009.

7

BROT UND SPIELE: EVOLUTION OF THE GDR

WE HAVE seen that the entire East German state doping system was nothing more than a means of using sport to enable a small European nation to establish itself on the international scene. In reality, this is not a completely new idea. Contrary to what was argued, a little hypocritically, by former IOC president Avery Brundage[187] ('Politics and sports should not mix. ... We deal with sports, not politics or business'),[188] since the time of the ancient Greeks, sport has always been considered a political resource, both from an external point of view, i.e. international relations, and from an internal one, as a phenomenon of aggregation among citizens. The history of the Olympic Games, just to mention the most important event, has always been studded with political and business interference. We are all well aware of certain corrupt phenomena that have plagued the decision to assign the organisation of the event, or the pressure that various sponsors exert in order to change local laws and regulations.[189]

We have seen great political boycotts, in 1980 (by the United States and 65 other nations) and in 1984 (by the USSR

---

187 In office from 1952 to 1972.

188 Mike Dennis, Jonathan Grix, *Sport Under Communism – Behind the East German Miracle*, Palgrave Macmillan, 2012.

189 Steven Walker, *Festival of Profits: Olympic traditions of capitalism and corruption continue*, peoplesworld.com, 10 June 2021.

and Warsaw Pact countries), violent episodes, such as the notorious 'bloodbath' at Melbourne 1956 between the USSR and Hungary water polo teams, and tragic events, such as the attack at Munich 1972 by the Palestinian terrorist group Black September. In other sport events, we have even witnessed surreal scenes, such as the one that happened in Chile, in 1973: because of a recent military coup, the Soviet Union team refused to travel to South America to take part in the play-off for the 1974 World Cup in Germany; so, the game was played, but with only Chile's footballers on the pitch, scoring goals without an opponent.

In 1974, the GDR national football team threatened not to play a World Cup match because it was to be held in West Berlin, a city still under the influence of the USA, UK and France, and boycotted by the Eastern Bloc. Intensive diplomatic work was necessary to unlock the stalemate and allow the *Fußballnationalmannschaft* to play their match against Chile. Again in Chile, Italian tennis players initially refused to go and play the Davis Cup Final in 1976 – the sports complex had been used as a concentration camp during the coup. After a lengthy political debate, the *Azzurri* decided to go, but they chose to wear 'socialist red' shirts (instead of the classic blue) during the games, as a mark of protest against the Pinochet regime. The list of similar events could go on: the bitter and realistic conclusion is that politics has often affected sport and vice versa.

Preparing for big sports events almost always has enormous costs for the community of the organising country, but local politicians are always happy to sacrifice economic resources on the altar of glory. For example, the 1976 Montréal Olympics caused a $3 billion debt to the province of Quebec; a debt that the Canadian people only finished paying in 2006![190]

---

190 Mark Johnson, *Spitting in the Soup: Inside the Dirty Game of Doping in Sports*, 2006.

In 2010, India, a developing country seeking to impose itself on the world scene, took on the burden of organising the Commonwealth Games, at the exorbitant cost of $4 billion; evidently, the New Delhi government felt it was more important to promote sporting events rather than solve other long-standing problems in a country where most people live in poverty.[191] In Italy, the municipality of Rome has yet to complete the payment of one billion euro, dating back to the 1960 Olympics![192] Contrary to what Brundage proclaimed, there is indeed no sport without politics.

No matter the cost, investing in sports has always been a viable method of putting a country on the map. In order to achieve that goal, at some point in its history the German Democratic Republic decided to invest large sums of money in sport; its politicians understood that sport is not just games or entertainment, but also, and above all, a formidable vehicle for propagating the cultural values of a society to other nations. According to the guidelines of the East German elite, sport strengthens the feeling of belonging of an individual as part of the team (and, by extension, of the society in which he lives): in fact, physical activities and competitions have the merit of uniting large fronds of the population in a transversal manner, regardless of the citizen's religious, cultural or economic background. Sports minister Manfred Ewald was convinced that physical activity is certainly an emotional release valve at a relatively low cost and promotes the well-being of those who practise it. Sport also facilitates the development of skills that are particularly useful for social purposes, such as teamwork, cooperation, motor activity, alertness, willpower, endurance and efficiency: all components that help in creating a healthier, more motivated and energetic society, in perfect

---

191 Jacquelin Magnay, *Commonwealth Games 2010 costs ballooned to over $4bn*, The Telegraph, 5 August 2011.

192 Ernesto Menicucci, *Raggi: «Le Olimpiadi nel 2024? Pesa ancora il debito del '60»*, Corriere della Sera, 16 August 2016.

harmony with the ideals of the socialist individual. Socialism, therefore, would find its glorification not only in the athletes' performances, but in the positive and purposeful behaviour of its citizens.[193]

To further confirm its importance, the term 'sport' is mentioned in at least four articles of the constitution of the German Democratic Republic. In particular, Article 34 promotes sport as a 'right of the individual', on a par with freedom of speech, religion and association – that some of these rights were then disregarded in real life is another matter. In short, sport had all the right characteristics to be used for political purposes to promote the image of a young nation like the GDR abroad and increase its international prestige.[194]

In 1948, the future head of state, Erich Honecker, then leader of the Free Youth Movement (FDJ), said: 'Sport is not an end, but the means to an end.'[195] Could there have been more prophetic words than these? The much-coveted recognition ('the end') would materialise during the 1970s and 80s, at the most important sport events.

Birth of a prodigious sports system

How did East Germany succeed in creating one of the most powerful and efficient sports systems in the world? It is evident that doping alone could never have produced the amazing sportsmen and sportswomen we have seen so many times on the podium celebrating record-breaking performances. There must have been more.

---

193 Manfred Ewald, *Körperkultur und Sport sind Sache unseres ganzen Volkes*, Theorie und Praxis der Körperkultur, 23, 1974.

194 J. Riordan, *The Impact of Communism on Sport*, The International Politics of Sport in the Twentieth Century, Spon Press, 1999.

195 G. Hotzweissig, *Die Funktion des Sports für das Herrschaftssystem der DDR*, Deutscher Bundestag, 1995.

Let's start from the beginning. After the Second World War, the Allies had divided the German territory into four zones of influence: three sectors in the west, ruled by France, the United States and Great Britain and one in the east, controlled by the Soviet Union. In the new nascent state of the Democratic Republic, East German citizens wanted, as far as possible, to go back to normal life: the launch of a national sports programme was one of the ideas that could give a sense of self-determination to people, but before taking any decision, the government had to deal first with the policies and interference of the Russian leader, Stalin. It took about three years and a lot of diplomacy before the new-born socialist state was given permission to start a real, autonomous sports plan; this was considered, by the East German government, indispensable for the development of social cohesion and for the affirmation of a national identity.

After several attempts, the first concrete act was to bring together all the then independent sports clubs under a single system of state control. The brain behind the project was Walter Ulbricht, a former leader of the German Communist Party, exiled to Moscow during the Third Reich period, and returned to Germany after the war. A sports enthusiast and a ski, tennis and volleyball practitioner, in the 1950s he started a strong campaign to promote the values of sport and its benefits for body and mind. When Ulbricht held the office of secretary of the SED, the Socialist Party, in the 50s and then became head of state, from 1960 to 1973, he gave further impetus to the process of nationalisation and centralisation of the sports system, managing to attain levels of efficiency that were, all in all, unexpected for a nation recovering from a devastating war and, in any case, subject to constant interference from the Soviet Union. The key points included: the politicisation of all sports disciplines; the distribution of benefits and privileges to the best athletes and coaches; the creation of dozens of Youth Sports Centres (KJS); the introduction of sophisticated programmes for preparing world-class coaches and developing elite sports centres (known as sports clubs, SC) in which to welcome the most promising athletes who could compete at international level. The very first centres to emerge were Motor Jena, Dynamo Berlin and Wissenschaft DHfK; initially, the main activities were football, handball, athletics and boxing. The most immediate objective of the sports programme was to match and (possibly) exceed the performances of, at least, the West German athletes. Even the clubs' names no longer echoed the imperialist matrix typical of their Western counterparts, but tried to represent the new socialist-Marxist trend of Soviet nature; names such as *Concordia* or *Borussia* were replaced by *Aktivist*, *Traktor* or *Dynamo*.

The 'female factor' was particularly important. Doctors and trainers realised that most foreign countries did not have many women in their Olympic teams; it was thus decided to take advantage of this lack of female athletes on the international scene, by trying to promote the recruitment of young East German girls, in addition to the usual enrolment of boys. Apart from the usual 'sprint' disciplines, the GDR coaches had the intuition to train the girls in power and endurance sports as well: at that time, these disciplines were exclusively for boys, but they would soon be opened to female contestants. This choice bore a strong political connotation, in the wake of the socialist principle of equality between men and women.[196] Positive results arrived soon. As early as the mid-1950s, hurdler Gisela Köhler and sprinter Christa Stubnick were able to attain world-level performances during national sports events.

Unfortunately for East Germany, the recognition of its own National Olympic Committee was slow in coming; its

---

196 G. Pfister, *Frauen und Sport in der DDR*, Sport und Buch Strauss, 2002.

approval was often the cause of heated discussions among the members of the IOC, mainly in consideration of the fact that the Republic had not yet been recognised by the international community as a country in its own right. After a series of discussions, boycotts, dropouts, proposals and cross-vetoes by various nations, East German athletes were allowed to participate in the 1952 Helsinki Olympics together with those from West Germany, in a single Olympic team. The GDR leaders did not take it well and, in protest, they refused to send their athletes to Finland.

During the first years of the Cold War, a feeling of opposition was increasingly developing between the two Germanic peoples. Despite the fact that both East and West Germans had origins and cultural traditions in common, the influences of the Allied countries, victors of the war, had given rise to various differences, in social and political terms, between them. These diversities widened more and more over the years, due to the different ideological paths of the two nations: the pro-NATO capitalist principles of West Germany on the one hand, against the pro-Soviet socialist principles of East Germany, on the other. The reciprocal and constant propaganda mechanisms, that prompted both countries to praise their ideology as 'better than the other one', led to an increasingly bitter rivalry between them. In general, West Germany, advocate of consumerism and gradually more accustomed to a certain well-being, experienced a decisive period of growth during the 50s in various sectors, such as industry, agriculture and social and economic development, whilst East Germany always lagged behind.

Focusing on the sports field, the main difference between the two nations was expressed in their ideological conception: as historian Ulrich Pabst points out, 'The Federal Republic wanted a sport without the influence of politics, whilst the Democratic Republic, on the contrary, desired its total politicisation.'[197] West German citizens still remembered the disturbing sport-political connection that was promoted by the Nazi regime (evocatively represented in the film *Olympia* by director Leni Riefenstahl), with all the negative aspects, in terms of Aryan propaganda and anti-Semitism, that had ensued at the 1936 Berlin Olympics, and they did not want the government to exploit their athletes' wins for political ends. On the other hand, the East Germans wasted no time in putting sport at the service of politics and in tying it inextricably to the values of socialism: the athletes' victories would bestow immediate prestige on the government, its leaders and the entire people of the GDR.

Of course, within East Germany, sport was also used as a distraction from the problems of everyday life. The always valid adage 'bread and circuses' was applied by the SED leaders to a mass of citizens whose socio-economic conditions were certainly not as prosperous as those who lived on the other side of the Iron Curtain. In any case, there was no shortage of work and entertainment. Basically, what interested the leaders of the state was to achieve the control of the masses, regardless of whether they really believed in the values of socialism or not. Those who accepted the status quo without complaining could even lead a comfortable life, albeit modest and with limited intellectual initiatives.[198] For a population that had just emerged from the ashes of the Second World War, it was out of the question to get involved in class struggles and cultural revolutions that would only bring people back to the conditions of 1945.

In light of an increasingly bitter ideological conflict between the two Germanys, it was obvious that the primary objective of the Socialist Party's leaders was to excel in all

---

197 Ulrich Pabst, *Sport-Medium der Politik?*, Verlag Bartels & Wemitz KG, 1980.

198 De Bruyn, *Jubelschreie, Trauergesange, Deutsche Befindlichkeiten*, Fischer Verlag, 1994.

sports, especially against their Western neighbours. It was important to show that a country of frugal socialist workers and amateur athletes was stronger and more deserving than a country of professional athletes, ruled by 'corrupt capitalists'. In reality, even if they were not professionals, the GDR athletes used to receive cash prizes for the results attained during major sporting events. Naturally, these were off-the-book payments. The first athlete to receive these fees was Herbert Friedel, the ski jumping world champion, who in 1951 received the not modest sum of 2,000 marks. The practice lasted for 40 years and was also confirmed by Ruth Fuchs, javelin legend and parliamentarian after the reunification of 1990: 'The money was often given by hand, stealthily and anonymously, by someone who slipped it into an envelope, in the mailbox.'[199]

Meanwhile, in 1955, West Germany promulgated the Hallstein Doctrine (named after the foreign minister who had conceived it), according to which the recognition of the GDR as an independent state by a foreign country, was to be considered a hostile act. For many years, West Germany was in fact the nation that most opposed any proposal to accept the existence of the German Democratic Republic, both as a nation-state and as a sporting entity. After much debate, for the 1956 Melbourne Olympics a compromise was finally found: the athletes of the two Germanys would compete under a neutral flag (the typical German one, but with the addition of the five Olympic rings). Of the 158 athletes of the United Germany delegation, 37 came from the GDR: among their athletes who stood out were Wolfgang Behrendt, Klaus Richtzenhain, Christa Stubnick, Gisela Köhler, Eva-Maria ten Elsen and renowned cyclist Gustav Schur. The latter became one of the most popular East German sportsmen ever. After winning the amateur World Championship twice, on

---

199 Ruth Fuchs e Klaus Ullbrich, *Lorbeerkranz und Trauerflor: Aufstieg und 'Untergang' des Sport wunders DDR*, Dietz Verlag, 1990.

the third occasion he clearly let team-mate Eckstein pass (and win) near the finish line, creating the myth of the gentleman cyclist. Amidst Olympic medals and acts of sporting generosity, the Ulbricht policy was beginning to bear fruit.

In 1957, in the wake of the positive enthusiasm arising from the Australian Games, the East German government decided to leap forward and create one of the most colossal sports organisations in Europe: the German Federation of Sports and Gymnastics (DTSB). This institute was conceived by men of the SED, but over time it became an independent entity, beyond the control of any government body. About half of the GDR members of parliament were also active associates of the DTSB; this combination, the only one of its kind in the world, guaranteed almost unlimited funds.

The DTSB was ubiquitous throughout the nation; in its organisation chart it included sports structures that were headed by various state bodies such as agricultural collectives, the army, universities, the police and internal security agents; each of them had their own sports club, and were often in bitter competition with each other. In its first year of life, the DTSB could already count 1.4 million members. In 1989, right before the end of the GDR, there were 3.7 million members – about 22 per cent of the population practised sport of some kind.[200]

The 'assembly line' for the recruitment of athletes had a pyramid structure; this was implemented through an original method, called ESA (*Einheitiliche Sichtung und Auswahl* – Uniform Monitoring and Selection), which was set up to help identify young talents from pre-adolescent age. The GDR, in fact, was keen to make up for the relatively low number (compared to other equally advanced nations) of citizens, which was about 17 million; each teenager therefore had to

200 Mike Dennis and Jonathan Grix, *Sport Under Communism – Behind the East German Miracle*, Palgrave Macmillan, 2012.

be tested to see if they had the potential to, one day, compete internationally. The search criteria for the 'champion of the future' were strictly scientific, to the point that it was possible to predict a probable sporting career for 10 to 12-year-old children, using complex algorithms.

The ESA method involved a series of measurements of various physical characteristics of the children (weight, height, limb length, particular sport inclination, etc.) to be carried out in their first, fourth and eighth school year. Boys and girls were tested in various disciplines: 60m sprint competitions, rope jumping, long jump, seven-minute endurance run and shot put. Motor activity, in general, and the ability to play as a team were also checked. All students able to perform within certain parameters or limits were considered for a possible sport career. For example, the minimum qualification for a 3,000m run was 12 minutes and 10 seconds for a 14-year-old boy, 11 minutes and 45 seconds for a 15-year-old boy, and 11 minutes and 33 seconds for a 16-year-old boy.[201]

Once the children were accepted in the sports centres or sports clubs, a further important step was necessary: an interview with the parents. Contrary to what one might think, even a dictatorial state like that of East Germany could not compel children to pursue an elite sports career without the consent of their families. East German coaches knew that performance in sport is, in fact, closely linked with the psychological condition of the athlete – an unhappy athlete will never achieve world-class results. The somewhat uncompromising approach of the early years soon had to soften because of the complaints of many parents, who were often even denied a visit to their children. The sports clubs' executives eventually gave way to a more flexible management of students, in mutual

---

201 Mike Dennis and Jonathan Grix, *Sport Under Communism – Behind the East German Miracle*, Palgrave Macmillan, 2012.

agreement with children and family members – at times, the students' prolonged isolation from their loved ones had caused them to abandon sports and a viable compromise had to be established. Even the dreaded *Stasi* understood how essential it was to talk with the parents and convince them that their children would be well cared for and trained, if they did not want to risk losing years of investment in the younger generation of athletes. Of course, as we have seen in the previous chapters, there would also be episodes of coercion, cruelty and blackmail.

Every year, 26,000 children aged between six and 15 were needed (depending on the sporting discipline) to fill the approximately 1,700 Youth Training Centres (TZ, the base of the pyramid) spread throughout the country: in these facilities, there were a total of about 67,000 children who trained three to five days a week, after school. From these centres, after three years of sacrifice, about 2,500 young people (aged 11–14) a year were promoted to one of the 25 Youth Sports Centres (KJS) located in the major cities of the East German territory. The training days were particularly hard: the boys who attended these centres spent about ten hours a day between sports and school subjects.[202] Of course, there were minimum requirements and goals to hit, in terms of distance, time or exercise, depending on the type of sport. Those who were not good enough to meet the standards were left out and had to give up their sports career. There are numerous testimonies of parents who, citing various excuses, asked the coaches to allow their children to repeat the tests. These second chances weren't generally granted, but sometimes, especially in schools in rural areas, where the number of enrolments was chronically low, they tried to adopt more flexibility or perhaps direct unsuccessful athletes

---

202 Mike Dennis and Jonathan Grix, *Sport Under Communism – Behind the East German Miracle*, Palgrave Macmillan, 2012.

towards an alternative discipline where they could get better results.[203]

The best athletes were constantly supervised by a highly trained teaching staff; sports managers and teachers had been hired in large numbers, to the point that the ratio of coaches to students was about 1:6. In the KJS, in addition to studying traditional subjects, such as literature, mathematics and science, children were also indoctrinated to the political rules of the SED. A document from the *Stasi* archives reads: 'The entire process of teaching and learning in the KJS must be directed to the formation and development of socialist personalities.'[204] Access to the KJS was considered a great honour for an East German child and, consequently, for their family; attending these schools amounted to a notable climb up the social ladder.[205]

KJS students also had the opportunity to study traditional subjects – these would have been useful in obtaining a good professional occupation once their sports career was over. These young people were monitored very carefully in their educational and sporting paths, and if they needed more time for homework, this was usually granted. Compared to normal schools, the KJS lasted one year longer: the purpose was to combine traditional study and sport, without compromising either of them. Children were encouraged to keep a diary where they could record their progress with respect to training plans, and also to follow and write comments on their 'sports heroes'. These notes were often checked by their teachers, and if one of those 'heroes' had been an athlete from the Western Bloc, or from a country not in accordance with the principles of socialism, the page would be removed and the child scolded.

203 Ibid.

204 BStU, *MfS und Leistungssport. Ein Rechercheberich*, Reihe A, Dokumente 1.

205 Barbara Cole, *The East Germany Sports System: Image and Reality*, University of Texas, 2001.

Only the best young athletes were selected from the KJS schools; these would then go on to compete under the aegis of one of the approximately 40 civil or military sports clubs of the GDR (the top of the pyramid). They contained, in total, about 3,000 athletes: a very low number, if we compare it with the starting amount at the bottom of the pyramid (67,000); a sign that the selection process was particularly rigorous.[206]

The DTSB was the organisation that acted as a link between sports schools (from Berlin to the most remote locations) and the Ministry of Sports, and enjoyed a high level of management autonomy. In total, 35 sports federations were part of it. The first president was Rudi Reichert, followed in 1961 by Manfred Ewald, a very powerful individual and great promoter of the doping system, who remained in office until 1988.[207] Ewald was Erich Honecker's trusted lieutenant and was known to be a highly skilled, manipulative, and self-centred politician. He had had a rather adventurous life. Born in 1926 into a family of German communists, he joined the Hitler Youth organisation, with the intention of spying on their plans on behalf of the anti-Nazi resistance. He was eventually identified together with other young communists, and sentenced to death, but managed to save himself from being shot thanks to the intervention of a Nazi officer who knew him personally. At the end of the war, he immediately entered the ranks of the newly formed SED.[208] From 1973 to 1990, he also held the position of president of the East German Olympic Committee. The importance of Manfred Ewald in the East German sports management system can

206 H.J. Teichler, K. Reinartz, *Das Leistungssportsystem der DDR in den 80er Jahren und im Prozess der Wende*, Verlag Karl Hoffmann, 1999.

207 Mike Dennis, Jonathan Grix, *Sport Under Communism – Behind the East German Miracle*, Palgrave Macmillan, 2012.

208 Doug Gilbert, *The Miracle Machine*, Coward, McCann & Geoghegan, New York, 1980.

certainly be summed up by the title of his autobiography: *'I Was Sport'*.[209]

Ewald's plan for the physical development of all German children became the key to forging athletes who would one day become champions. The basic idea had been taken, incredibly, from the 'corrupt' American system. At the beginning of the 1960s, Walter Ulbricht had sent a group of specialists to visit some schools in the United States; German sports executives gathered that the successes of American gymnasts, sprinters and swimmers depended on the fact that from an early age they were educated in the culture of sacrifice and ambition.

One of the most interesting conclusions drawn by the study group was that the average American child was less educated than the German one; spending less time doing homework gave young people the opportunity to use that surplus time to train and participate in local competitions against other schools. Those students spent on average twice as long in the gym as their German peers and had the use of state-of-the-art sports equipment. The approach seemed the right one and was basically imported to East Germany, where it was soon studied, modified and improved. It was obvious that, in the long run, the country with the best recruitment system of young people would win the most medals.

The East German study group also discovered the American sports system's main weakness: the US coaches trained the children exclusively through their personal beliefs, ability and experience; the pool of young athletes in a certain community was therefore destined for success or oblivion depending on the methods of its coach. In East Germany, they thought it wasn't acceptable to leave the athletes' training to chance and decided to create the DHfK, the University of Physical Education: a unique structure of its kind, based in Leipzig, where all coaches would study and get prepared in

---

209 Manfred Ewald, *Ich War der Sport*, Elefanten Press, 1994.

the same way. Some of them could also reach very high levels of specialisation through the achievement of post-graduate research doctorates. The Leipzig study centre was at the forefront of the world, with 11 sports halls, athletics tracks and swimming pools, all strictly Olympic-sized. At the heart of the complex was a majestic 100,000-seat stadium.[210]

Advanced technology and well-prepared coaches were two important ingredients in building the perfect sport machine. A third one was needed and it had to be developed nearly from scratch: a sporting and winning mentality. In order to achieve this, sport was widely promoted in schools and workplaces. Even Manfred Ewald, as supreme head of sport in the GDR, enrolled in college in Leipzig, studied and took his coaching licence, a qualification which in East Germany had the rank of a degree. 'As president of the DTSB,' Ewald liked to emphasise, 'how could I make sports-related decisions, if I didn't have the right skills?'[211] For an in-depth look at the DHfK curriculum of study, please refer to Appendix III.

Regular contests between athletes of the same age were the key to accustom all children to the competitive atmosphere of sport events. In this regard, in 1966, the SED decided to organise the *Spartakiade*, a sort of student Olympics in which about 10,000 children would compete every two years. These games showed an organisational level worthy of a great event, complete with the participation of various party leaders, journalists from the most important newspapers and the young athletes' parents. The occasion was naturally used by the government to deliver propaganda speeches on the principles of socialism and to indoctrinate the students' minds. The *Spartakiade* was also used as a vehicle for political action.

---

210 *Zentralstadion*, today renamed Red Bull Arena. After the reunification, it hosted five matches during the 2006 FIFA World Cup.

211 Doug Gilbert, *The Miracle Machine*, Coward, McCann & Geoghegan, New York, 1980.

In 1966, for example, there was a great deal of emphasis on the 'dirty war in Vietnam', with fundraising to help the war-torn populations of South-east Asia.[212]

The investments were considerable: in the period 1967–70 the sport-dedicated funds increased from 5.5 million marks to 16 million! It was now clear to the government that it would be complicated to affirm their nation abroad in the fields of trade, politics and culture; the only possibility of obtaining some respect from the international community was through the achievement of extraordinary sport results.

However, the distribution of funding was not the same for all; two categories had been created within the DTSB, called Sport I and Sport II, which would have different federations grouped according to their chances of winning medals and that, consequently, would receive different amounts of money. The Sport I group included the following associations: athletics, football, swimming, boxing, fencing, weightlifting, handball, judo, canoeing, cycling, wrestling, rowing, shooting, diving, sailing, gymnastics, volleyball, biathlon, skating, bobsleigh and skiing. These sports could count on substantial funding and also on adequate organisation to enable them to participate in major events.

All other federations belonged to the Sport II group; this included horse riding, basketball, tennis and hockey. They received such limited funds that they could not even properly finance their participation in the Olympics; over time, this inequality of treatment would widen more and more, leading to the dissolution of many gyms and the firing of coaches and managers. Over the years, the discrepancy between funding for mass sports and for the elite sports clubs would be amplified: the latter would grab most of it, creating discontent among amateur athletes and resentment against the government,

---

212 Barbara Cole, *The East Germany Sports System: Image and Reality*, University of Texas, 2001.

which, while inviting everyone to play sports, was not always able to guarantee adequate facilities and clothing.

In addition to financing technical structures and forging skilled managers, there was also a need to provide cash incentives to athletes. For example, for the 1988 Seoul Olympics, a 35,000-mark bonus was allocated to medal-winning athletes. To prevent some of them from suddenly withdrawing and running away with the money, the bonuses were delivered only at the end of the athletes' careers. There was also a series of privileges such as preferential access to *Intershops* (stores authorised to sell consumer goods from West Germany – small oases of Western consumerism within the GDR), as well as a spacious house and a good job.

It is therefore in this context of 'state interference' in all aspects of life, including sport, work and social activities, that the method of citizen control developed, together with the state doping system. The government was positively convinced that the people involved (doctors, coaches, managers and bureaucrats of all sorts) would gladly accept it, as we have clearly seen, patriotically and without asking too many questions.

Rise and recognition

Politically, the East German Olympic Committee was founded in 1951 but was only recognised by the IOC in 1965. In Europe, however, things were different: the GDR, which had obtained its status as an independent nation from the Soviet Union in 1955, received the authorisation to participate in continental tournaments almost immediately. Included in the most important events of this decade, were the European Athletics Championships in Stockholm (1958), where the GDR won six medals, and those in Belgrade four years later (eight medals). In swimming, East Germany's first international participation dates back to the 1954 European Championships in Turin, where they came third in the medal table. Subsequently, they took part in the European Championships in Budapest in 1958 (collecting only one bronze), and organised those of 1962, in Leipzig, where they collected five gold medals. Further recognition came from the *Union Cycliste Internationale*, when in 1960 they assigned the organisation of the Cycling World Championships to Karl-Marx-Stadt – it was the event at which Schur made his generous gesture, as we saw earlier.

In the rest of the world, apart from in gymnastics and football, the GDR was unable to attain the desired recognition. After acquiring the right to participate in the 1956 Olympics, as seen above, jointly with West Germany (a condition that also applied for Rome 1960 and Tokyo 1964, when the GDR athletes actually won more medals than the FRG athletes for the first time), in 1968 they were finally allowed to compete as a separate nation. There was a caveat, though: the communist symbols on the GDR flag had to be replaced by the Olympic rings, and Beethoven's 'Ode to Joy' was played instead of the official national anthem, the austere 'Auferstanden aus Ruinen',[213] (which would be heard hundreds of times during the awards ceremonies of major sport events from the 1970s onwards).

In the Olympic Games where East Germany and West Germany competed jointly, the copious GDR medals were overshadowed by the fact that the victories were 'collective', i.e. belonging to a united Germany, which frustrated the SED leaders immensely. The path that eventually led to the much-desired achievement of independence was decidedly tortuous, and not without episodes of boycott by the Bonn government. One of the most sensational and irritating incidents occurred in September 1965, when the DTSB president, Manfred Ewald, was denied access to West Berlin; the executive needed to cross the border temporarily to access the Spanish embassy

---

213 'Rising from the Ruins'.

and apply for a visa, in order to participate in the international meeting of the IOC in Madrid. That rejection prevented the GDR from being represented at the IOC assembly, creating a wider crack between the two nations. The East–West rift was not mended until a few years later, with the election of Willy Brandt as chancellor of the FRG, his policy of *détente* towards the East (*Ostpolitik*), and the consequent definitive rebuff of the Hallstein Doctrine.

As mentioned before, 1968 was the year in which East Germany could finally participate in all official international competitions separately from West Germany. The first important occasion was the Winter Olympics in Grenoble. That event, long awaited by the DTSB leaders, proved to be a tough test for the Eastern delegation from the point of view of image and diplomacy. Almost a month earlier, in fact, during a training camp in Switzerland, the East German skier Ralph Pohland had fled from the hotel where he was staying with his national team, and had managed to defect to West Germany, creating enormous embarrassment for his compatriots. Pohland succeeded thanks to an ingenious plan carried out with the complicity of Georg Thoma, a West German skier, a journalist from the ZDF[214] (who reported the event in the Western media) and the West German Ski Federation. The latter had prepared all the necessary documents for the change of nationality and promised Pohland that he would participate in the Olympics as a member of the FRG national team. The skier was deemed a traitor in his country and the *Stasi* took action, unsuccessfully, to bring him back. In order to convince the athlete to return to the GDR, the *Stasi* targeted his parents, who lost their jobs and were even arrested, but Ralph didn't change his mind. Unable to get him back, the East German government played the final card to save its reputation: during the Olympics, the GDR and the Soviet

---

214 *Zweites Deutsches Fernsehen*, a West Germany television channel.

Union delegations jointly asked the IOC to disqualify Pohland for unfair behaviour, threatening to withdraw their athletes from the Games if this did not happen. Despite the usual reassurances to the skier, in the end the Olympic Committee was forced to give in to the blackmail and to suspend Pohland from all competitions for six months.[215] From that moment on, the East German authorities would take exceptional measures to prevent any further attempt at defection. Perhaps because of that episode, the debut of the national team was not as good as expected, as they won just one gold medal, two silver and two bronze.

At the 1968 Mexico City Olympics (which turned out to be a great success, as GDR won nine gold medals and finished fifth in the medal table), all the athletes were subjected to a severe screening in which they had to attest their sense of political affiliation to the socialist ideology. Anyone who expressed any doubts about the directives of the Socialist Unity Party (SED) would be left at home, even at the cost of losing some important competitors. Did this party line work?

In her doctoral thesis, East German javelin thrower Ruth Fuchs researched, in the 1980s, the real motivation that pushed athletes to compete, concluding that the inspiration to do well for their country obviously came from a socialist ideological drive. No one seemed to put forward personal justifications, such as glory, fame, improvement of their social condition, or the chance to travel abroad. In a study by the Texan researcher Barbara Cole in the post-Wall period of the 1990s, more than 20 athletes declared that fidelity to the ideals of Marxism-Leninism was in fact the least important aspect that could provide inspiration.[216] Olympic swimmer Roland Matthes candidly confirms this conclusion: 'We knew

---

215 Jutta Braun, Michael Barsuhn, *Flucht zum Freund*, Der Tagesspiel, February 2008.

216 Barbara Cole, *The East Germany Sports System: Image and Reality*, University of Texas, 2001.

where we lived. These standards were part of the apparatus's *raison d'être*. In Erfurt, for example, the party secretary came into the swimming pool once and said: "Remember, what we are doing here is class warfare!" He may have believed that he had achieved something, that he had given the trainer direction. That, of course, was absurd! I did my best in the water for myself and for my coach, and then for my club. I don't know of any athletes, really none, who did it solely for the state.'[217] Evidently, during the years of the Republic, athletes had realised that it was more convenient for their lives and their careers to try to grin and bear it.

The socialist principles were, however, very much present and dominated the athletes' lives; willingly or unwillingly, they had to behave according to the ideology imposed by the SED. Consequently, disciplinary action was taken against those athletes who did not align with the dictates of socialist thought. During the 1966 European Athletics Championships in Budapest, for instance, East German runner Jürgen Haase, after winning the 10,000m race, was approached by Jürgen May, a team-mate, who suggested he wear Puma shoes instead of the officially approved Adidas ones, in the upcoming 5,000m race. May had received $100 from Puma and was tasked with giving Haase $500, should he agree to run in the new shoes. When a vigilant executive of the East German Athletics Federation realised that Haase was wearing different shoes, he asked the runner why. He immediately confessed the agreement with Puma and handed the money (and the shoes) over to the manager. An investigation followed: May was disqualified for life for having succumbed to the lure of capitalism, while Haase, given his young age, was pardoned. May became *persona non grata* and, thanks to the intercession of some Puma executives,

---

217 Grit Hartmann, *Goldkinder*, Forum Verlag Leipzig, 1998.

he was allowed to migrate to West Germany.[218] Evidently, it was important for the GDR government to send a message to all athletes to enforce the rules and principles of socialism and not be duped by the sirens of capitalism. There was, in fact, a concrete fear that reports coming through Western radios and televisions, which most East Germans were able to receive in their homes, could negatively affect the impressionable minds of the young athletes.

Of course, over time, the GDR executives eventually had to bow to plutocracy principles, when they entered into a lucrative sponsorship agreement with Adidas (a multinational corporation based in despised West Germany) for the remarkable sum of 500,000 marks for the right to supply shoes, overalls and various accessories, plus an extra 1.5 million marks per year.[219] In that instance, the GDR leaders proved to be particularly accustomed to commercial negotiations. Even in East Germany, at the right moment, the old saying *pecunia non olet*[220] could apply.

Explosion and dominion

When on 26 April, 1966, the IOC announced that Munich would host the 1972 Olympic Games, Manfred Ewald and all of the SED executives felt a mixture of alarm and elation; the future television reports produced by the West German channels would certainly be seen by their fellow citizens who lived in the areas close to the border (about 70 per cent of the entire population).[221] TV stations such as ARD and ZDF could

---

218 Adolf Metzner, *Der Krieg der Schuhe*, Die Zeit, 3 February 1967.

219 Mike Dennis, Jonathan Grix, *Sport Under Communism*, Palgrave MacMillan, 2012.

220 Money does not stink.

221 James M. Markham, *TV Brings Western Culture To East Germany*, The New York Times, 13 February 1984. (Only areas in the north-east and the south-east of the GDR weren't able to receive the 'Western' signal.)

show inconvenient information about their Western neighbours' lifestyles. Nevertheless, the event was also an incredible opportunity to make a good impression in front of the world, right in the home of their 'rivals'. Preparing in the most efficient way (both from the counter-propaganda point of view and from that of competition) was a goal of the utmost urgency.

East Germany's sporting triumph exploded at the Sapporo Winter Olympics, where the national team collected 14 medals in total (even occupying the entire podium on two occasions: men's and women's luge), and finished in second place in the medal table, performing better than the United States and, above all, West Germany.

The 1972 Munich Olympics was the first Summer Games in which the German Democratic Republic took part as a fully fledged independent nation – in addition to a formal recognition by the Brandt government, political acceptance by the United Nations Organisation would soon follow. In Bavaria, the GDR athletes won 20 gold medals, 23 silver medals and 23 bronze medals (getting third place overall in the medal table), in 18 different disciplines. The pompous Eastern leaders were able to enjoy the fact that the West German organisers had to hoist the East German flag 20 times, while the military band played their anthem. Willy Brandt, an advocate of *détente*, in a careless attempt to bring the two Germanys closer together, declared: 'If the GDR win medals, then we too win with them.'[222] The sentence greatly irritated the East German sports managers and they 'sent the message back to the sender'; they probably felt that by sharing their medals, even theoretically, their wins would lose the socialist connotations they promoted so much. However, the success of East Germany, together with that of the Soviets and other Eastern European athletes, was considered by the SED a

---

222 Hartmut Becker, *Der Olympische Aufstieg der DDR: Meinungsum-fragen in der Bundesrepublik*, Deutschland Archiv, 7, n.2, 1974.

triumph for the Eastern Bloc and their socialist ideology over Atlantic imperialism.

Obviously, staying in West Germany for two weeks would expose the East German athletes to the Western lifestyle; this couldn't be entirely avoided but could be minimised. Before the GDR delegation left for Munich, the East Berlin government prepared a 35-minute video that summarised the ideology of socialism, the dangers of consumerism and capitalism, and the beauty of East Germany – a sort of accelerated indoctrination course, or refresher lesson, conceived precisely to prevent athletes from being influenced by Western ways of life. Those who weren't members of the socialist party were severely scrutinised to test their loyalty before leaving the country. For instance, cyclist Wolfgang Lötzsch was excluded from the Munich squad due to political concerns after his cousin fled to the West; the fact that Lötzsch didn't want to become a member of the SED didn't help his cause. After submitting several applications to leave the country and openly supporting a dissident, he was even arrested in 1976.[223]

The athletes weren't allowed to walk the streets of Munich, remaining practically segregated inside the Olympic village. The only moment of allowable 'leisure' was a visit, obviously escorted, to the Dachau concentration camp! The danger of someone deciding to defect was always real; for this reason, the members of the Olympic delegation, and the fans, had to travel without wives or relatives with them: if anyone had planned to flee to the West, they would have had to leave their loved ones in East Germany.[224]

The controversies between the two Germanys continued throughout the period of the Summer Games. The two countries often exchanged press releases where they never

---

223 Wolfgang Lötzsch page in *ddr.zeitzeugen.de*
224 Barbara Cole, *The East Germany Sports System: Image and Reality*, University of Texas, 2001.

missed an opportunity to exalt their virtues and demonise the vices of the other, on the other side of the Wall. Even during the tragic terrorist attack by the Palestinian commandos, Black September, who kidnapped and subsequently killed ten Israeli athletes, there was little cooperation. Manfred Ewald refused, at least initially, to vacate the apartments occupied by the GDR athletes, a measure that would have allowed the police to control the hostage situation. Essentially, Ewald didn't want to run the risk of being accused of collaborating with the Western authorities. After hours of negotiations, the GDR official finally gave the order to his athletes to vacate the apartments and allow the police in.[225]

When the Olympic cauldron's flame at the Olympiastadion went out, the East German executives reaped the rewards of their investments: in the eyes of the world, East Germany finally appeared as a model of efficiency and discipline, capable of creating a technologically advanced centre of excellence for their young generations. The Olympic success was also celebrated by the SED leaders as 'a promotion of those socialist values, which go hand in hand with the physical and mental development of the individual'.[226]

At the following Winter Games in Innsbruck (1976), East German athletes further increased their tally of medals, winning 19 (including seven gold – more than the USA and West Germany together), placing themselves immediately behind the USSR in the medal table. The excellent result at the Austrian Games was the prelude to the triumph in Montréal, where the East German delegation far exceeded the expectations of all sports experts, winning 40 gold medals and finishing in second place in the medal table, right behind the

---

225 Serge Groussard, *The Blood of Israel: The Massacre of the Israel Athletes*, William Morrow and co., 1975.

226 G. Witt, *Mass Participation and Top Performance in One: Physical Culture and Sport in the German Democratic Republic*, The Journal of Popular Culture, 1984.

Soviet Union. It would be the event that saw the rise of Kornelia Ender, a star who dominated swimming competitions, and the first true East German athlete to achieve international media prominence. The Canadian Summer Olympics also provided a significant test bed for the *Stasi* security system, as many East German athletes travelled to American continental territory, exposed to all sorts of anti-communist propaganda and temptations of defection.

Former athlete Sigurd Hanke confirms how unhappy some of his fellow citizens were with the GDR regime, so much so that they could have taken advantage of their travels to leave the country. 'Yes, many people were dissatisfied. Many didn't even want to leave permanently, but at least wanted to be able to travel and see the alternatives to the Eastern Bloc. It is always a smaller part of the population that would actually emigrate. We humans are very attached to our homeland. I mean, that applies to all peoples, at all times. Even I thought about leaving the GDR. The more often I went to non-socialist countries and the older I got, the more [I thought it]. Why didn't I do it? I already had a girlfriend; according to the assessment at the time, we would never have seen each other again. My parents and my sister, also my girlfriend (now wife) would have experienced serious disadvantages and reprisals.'[227] Retaliation towards relatives was always a powerful incentive to dissuade athletes from defecting. However, the government knew that some of them could be well motivated and still try to flee to the West. Other than blackmail, a great deal of surveillance was required.

In order to efficiently control its athletes, the Ministry for State Security made every effort to ensure that among the accompanying staff of the Olympic delegation there were agents of the *Stasi*: out of 511 athletes, 67 were actually IM, informants of the intelligence services. Social interactions with

---

227 Correspondence with the author.

foreign athletes had to be kept to a minimum and, if allowed, they were always under close surveillance.[228] However, contacts with athletes from other nations were actually sought by the East Germans themselves when the situation allowed it, but it was absolutely vital not to be caught by their controllers: any hint of dialogue with people from other countries could be severely punished. For instance, a few years earlier, Andreas Kunz, skier and room-mate of the aforementioned defector Ralph Pohland, had been welcomed home like a hero for winning a bronze and for having stigmatised his colleague's escape. A few months later, however, the two were caught chatting while waiting to compete before a Ski World Cup race. Kunz was immediately sent back to East Berlin and accused of treason for having talked to the enemy.[229]

In some situations during training or competitions, away from prying eyes – not even the *Stasi* agents could be everywhere, especially in a foreign land – it was possible to chat, as reported by marathon runner Waldemar Cierpinski ('There were occasions to talk, but my problem was that I didn't speak English and I couldn't say much') and shot putter Udo Beyer ('I spent a lot of time with American colleagues to the point that I even learned to speak a little English'). Others could have attempted to socialise but for fear of retaliation they didn't even try.[230] Canoeist Kordula Striepecke clearly and comprehensively expresses the anguish of those moments in which she tried to fraternise with other athletes: 'We were in Mezzana, Italy, for a World Cup competition. We were banned from talking to other athletes, especially West Germans and Austrians. One day, during a lunch in the

---

228 The Canadian Press, *Stasi dumped syringes in St Lawrence in 1976*, CBC, 2009.

229 Jutta Braun, Michael Barsuhn, *Flucht zum Freund*, Der Tagesspiel, February 2008.

230 Barbara Cole, *The East Germany Sports System: Image and Reality*, University of Texas, 2001.

canteen, a Swiss athlete came to sit next to me and a colleague of mine. The first thing he asked us was something about the last elections in East Germany and whether they had been rigged. Panic! My team-mate was a member of the SED and I should have weighed my words well. I said that probably a 99.9 per cent vote result for Honecker was a bit exaggerated. Then I hastily added that if one of our coaches approached the table, we would have to leave, and that he shouldn't be offended by that move. Soon after, as expected, our coach joined us and we had to leave the table. A few hours later, that Swiss canoeist met us and thanked us for specifying the reason for our antisocial behaviour.'[231]

As ever, fear was the best way to convince the East German athletes not to start any kind of conversation with foreign delegates. The oppressive regime, so efficiently in action in their own country, used to be 'exported' to foreign soil during sport events. Considering that, in any year, the GDR team took part in many international competitions, the effort to minimise social interactions between the East Germans and the others must have been quite a remarkable feat.

Triumphs and boycotts

Surveillance issues were obviously expected four years later, at the 1980 Winter Olympics in Lake Placid, USA. However, in that situation, controlling the Olympic delegation would be simpler than it had been in Canada; Lake Placid is in fact a rather remote location in the hinterland of New York State, and the risks of the GDR athletes mingling with the local population, or coming into contact with the American lifestyle, were minimal. The sports results, once again, were outstanding. East Germany won nine gold medals, just one less than the USSR, but secured a greater overall total (23

---

231 Interview by John Paul Kleiner on his website (abridged version), *The GDR Objectified.*

medals against the USSR's 22 and the USA's 12). In addition to a performance below expectations, the United States didn't even shine from an organisational point of view: there were delays in transportation, long queues for the accreditation of journalists, insufficient hotel facilities for fans and even problems in the distribution of food. The Olympic village didn't look particularly welcoming as it was built in such a way that it would later be used as a federal prison. Not the best display, especially considering the fact that within a few months the Summer Olympics would be held in the heart of the Soviet Union.[232]

However, the Americans were not able to make comparisons between their own organisation and the Soviet one, in Moscow. As a mark of protest against the USSR's invasion of Afghanistan, which took place in 1979, the USA boycotted the Games on Russian soil. Initially, the US Secretary of State, Cyrus Vance, had asked the IOC to move the Olympics to another country, but the chairman of the committee, Lord Killanin, opposed the idea. At that point, the US President, Jimmy Carter, sent an ultimatum, calling for the withdrawal of Soviet troops from Afghanistan by 20 January 1980, otherwise the United States would not take part in the Games. Eventually, the American athletes stayed home.

In addition to the USA, for various reasons, as many as 65 countries refused to send their delegations to Moscow. Some European members of NATO decided to participate, but under the five-ring Olympic flag, and without their national anthem if they won gold. The absence of many countries obviously created an imbalance in the number of victories, all in favour of the Soviet Union (80 gold medals) and East Germany (47). Naturally, the success at the Moscow Olympics was hailed by the SED as a triumph of the Eastern

---

232 Barbara Cole, *The East Germany Sports System: Image and Reality*, University of Texas, 2001.

Bloc's socialist values of peace and coexistence against the despondent imperialism of the uninspiring Western Bloc.[233]

Bragging aside, East Germany had by now proved to be among the leading nations in the world of sports and was really beginning to gather support and admiration from the Western media as well. After Moscow, the renowned American magazine *Runner's World*, through reporter Brian Chapman, published a long article praising the scientific approach conceived by German doctors for long-distance disciplines; the use of sophisticated cameras, computerised analyses and high-tech equipment (such as hyperbaric chambers to simulate high-altitude environments, and counter-current swimming channels) calibrated by biomechanical engineers, were 'revolutionary innovations' that could not be found in other countries.[234] The weekly magazine *Newsweek* also pointed out that East German research methods were efficiently applied to sport, and the studies on the progress of athletes under laboratory conditions were an example to follow.[235]

The French journalist Paul Katz, while admitting the possibility that a certain form of doping could circulate among the East German athletes, praised the recruiting system to build 'champions of the future' from a very young age. Even the West Germans were interested in that system and did everything to steal its secrets through the various athletes who, from time to time, managed to escape from the GDR.[236] However, the most detailed and celebratory account in the

---

233 Norbert Lehmann, *Internationale Sportbeziehungen und Sportplitik der DDR*.
Tell I., Mimster: Lh. Verlag, 1986.

234 Brian Chapman, *'East of the Wall: East Germany training is aimed at Moscow 1980'*, Runner's World, March 1978.

235 Pete Axhelm and Frederick Kempe, *'The East German Machine'*, Newsweek, July 1980.

236 Paul Katz, *'East Germany Olympic Secrets: Muscle Culture Becomes an Exact Science'*, L'Express, April 1977.

Western world was the book *The Miracle Machine* by Doug Gilbert, a Canadian journalist whose incredible story has been told in the previous chapter.

After a few years of testing, the East German Olympic Committee (NOK) concluded that, in order to maximise the investment/medal ratio (i.e. obtaining the maximum number of victories with a lesser economic effort), it made sense to concentrate funding and resources on individual sports rather than team sports. In fact, it soon became obvious that coaching a hockey, basketball or water polo team cost a lot due to the large number of athletes involved and, in the end, a possible victory would only bring one medal.

In light of this new policy, at the Sarajevo Winter Olympics, in 1984, the only teams that the *Nationales Olympisches Komitee der DDR* decided to send were bobsleigh and luge; maximum participation was obviously guaranteed for all individual competitions. The strategy paid off, given that East Germany, for the first (and last) time in the history of the Olympics, managed to finish at the top of the table, with nine gold medals (ahead of the Soviet Union, six gold) and 24 in total. A total triumph! The Sarajevo Games marked the debut of the charismatic figure skater Katarina Witt, whose skill and physical beauty was also exalted by the Western media – the American magazine *Time* dedicated one of its covers to Witt, calling her 'The most beautiful face of socialism'. The skater drew so much attention that the *Stasi* feared a possible defection. Actually, Witt, who was not even a member of the SED, would always be loyal and grateful to her country, praising its organisational skills, even many years after the fall of the Wall.[237]

The months that separated the Olympics in Yugoslavia from those in Los Angeles were marked by a growing tension

---

237 Barbara Cole, *The East Germany Sports System: Image and Reality*, University of Texas, 2001.

between Eastern and Western Bloc countries. American President Ronald Reagan did everything to exploit the Olympic event for electoral purposes, focusing the campaign for his re-election on a classic Cold War topic: the danger of communism, as a toxic exhalation of the so-called 'Empire of Evil'. The rhetoric of the election campaign went beyond the US borders, invading the international field of political confrontation between the two great superpowers. In April 1984, the USSR formally asked the IOC to convene an urgent session to discuss Reagan's anti-communist propaganda. The USA were accused of displaying abusive diplomatic behaviour, especially after denying some Soviet Olympic representatives access to their country, on the grounds that they might be KGB agents. Furthermore, the Americans were considered guilty of having developed the idea of commercialising the Olympic Games, and downgrading their amateur aspect, through the inclusion of numerous official sponsors.[238]

The International Olympic Committee, which had approved the sponsorships, could not, of course, interfere with American domestic politics, and turned a deaf ear. The Brezhnev government, for security reasons and to protect its athletes from engaging 'in hostile territory and with strong anti-communist sentiments', decided not to send a delegation to Los Angeles.[239] To many commentators of the time, the withdrawal of the USSR actually seemed like an excuse to take revenge on the American boycott of four years earlier. East Germany and the other nations of the Warsaw Pact (except Romania, at the time in contrast with the Soviet leaders) also decided not to participate in the US Olympics.

---

238 Norm Clarke, *'It's official: Sponsors help pay for Olympics'*, Associated Press, 7 April, 1984.

239 *1984: Moscow pulls out of US Olympics*, BBC News, 8 May 1984.

Although the official position of the East Germans on the boycott was in line with that dictated by the Soviet Union, internally things were different. The top executives of the NOK were actually greatly irritated by the Kremlin's decision. Both the GDR government, which had lost an opportunity to win more medals and consolidate its position as a leader in the world of sports, and the athletes, who had seen the chance to improve their social position (through long-awaited awards) evaporate after years of training, later agreed in condemning their forced desertion from the Olympic dream. Ernst Schmickler, an executive of the East German National Radio, issued a statement, which in normal times would have resulted in sanctions (even heavy ones), blaming the Soviet authorities. He underlined the fact that the compulsory boycott imposed on the countries of the Eastern Bloc risked causing a deterioration in the relationship of trust with the Soviet sports authority: because of that decision, the athletes could develop a dangerous feeling of enmity towards the USSR. Finally, contrary to the Russian dictates, the East German media gave generous coverage to the Olympics, even in the absence of their athletes.[240] It was clear that Soviet interference in the GDR's plans had caused a laceration in the relations between the two countries; a tear that would continue to expand in the years to come.

Despite its absence from such an important event as the Olympics, the GDR still had the opportunity to stock up on medals at world and continental tournaments in various sports. Very often, East Germany ranked at the top of the medal table of those events. For those who experienced those incredible victories in front of a TV, like the writer of this book, the echo of the GDR national anthem was virtually ubiquitous, being performed at many awards ceremonies, to

240 Barbara Cole, *The East Germany Sports System: Image and Reality*, University of Texas, 2001.

the point of being redundant and even boring. That music had entered people's collective imagination so obsessively that the organisers of the 1985 Alpine Ski World Championships in Bormio erroneously played it to celebrate Markus Wasmeier's victory in the giant slalom event. The athlete was in fact a West German. The surprising thing is that the GDR was not even present at that event!

Crisis and epilogue

The anger at the forced exclusion from the Californian Games was saved and channelled into a strong determination to succeed at the Calgary Olympics in 1988. Despite the sporting enthusiasm, in those years East Germany was going through an economic crisis that called into question some of the strengths of its socialist political structure. Unemployment, for example, a phenomenon which up until then had been virtually non-existent, was beginning to manifest itself as a worrying reality. Prices to access entertainment facilities such as museums, cinemas and gyms, began to increase from their usually very low levels, creating some discontent among the population. East German athletes, who came into contact with the realities of Western capitalist welfare, began to wonder if the socialist system was, in fact, doomed to fail.

However, there was no lack of resources for elite sports: the athletes had all the technical and scientific support of the past years. In Calgary, they performed up to expectations, finishing in second place in the medal table, behind the USSR. Just like four years earlier, figure skater Katarina Witt was the star of the Games. However, her victory had a symbolic and material value that went beyond the gold medal. The athlete from Karl-Marx-Stadt had in fact managed to sign an unprecedented agreement with the East German government, in an attempt to open the door to professionalism for athletes from her country. The SED executives had promised her that if she managed to win gold in Calgary, they would give her the opportunity to go to the USA to take part in a three-year touring ice show, paired with Brian Boitano, a US Olympic skater. Witt triumphed in Canada and the GDR government kept its word. The ice show was very popular and sold out at many venues; the East German skater became the first GDR citizen to become a millionaire star; she would even win an Emmy Award for her performance in the movie *Carmen on Ice* (Horant Holfeld, 1990). By the end of the tour, the country where she had been born and raised would no longer exist.[241]

The 1988 Seoul Olympics gave the whole world a huge signal of *détente*, with the participation of the two great superpowers and their allies: in total, 159 nations took part. The GDR team achieved an excellent result, winning 37 gold medals and securing second position in the medal table behind the USSR. Swimmer Kristin Otto won six of those medals, setting a women's record which still stands. Otto, accused years later of doping, often protested her innocence. The swimmer pointed to the fact that the athletes' names were protected by a code at the Kreischa laboratory and that the connection between her name and the code has never been proven. Furthermore, she has not undergone the typical 'transformations' of doped athletes and her name has never been found on any *Stasi* lists.[242] After the Olympics, the Leipzig swimmer would have the opportunity to develop a successful career, graduating and becoming a sports journalist. Today, Kristin Otto is deputy director of sports services for ZDF, Germany's second-largest TV channel.

Seoul marked the final GDR participation at the Olympic Games.

After the feast of medals in South Korea, the problems of a fragile and regressive economy came to a head. More

241 Documentary *Katarina Witt – The Diva on Ice with a huge heart'* Legends Live On, Olympic Channel, 2018.
242 Werner Franke, *Kollektiver Zwang zum Schweigen*, Berliner Zeitung, 5 April 1994.

and more East German citizens started to complain about the constant unemployment growth, the deterioration of medical services, and the dire conditions of their dilapidated apartments. Resources for sport were also becoming scarce. The rise to power of the Soviet reformer Mikhail Gorbachev sent contradictory signals to the leading GDR politicians. His new policies of *Glasnost* (transparency) and *Perestroika* (reconstruction), which began the process of reforms that would lead to the dissolution of the Soviet Union within a couple of years, did not coincide with the dictates of isolationism and secrecy typical of East Germany. In order to give a strong signal of openness and relaxation, Gorbachev, at some point, suggested starting the 1989 edition of the *Friedensfahrt* (Peace Tour), a classic cycling race in stages that took place every year in Eastern Europe, in Paris. The route would have crossed France and the two Germanys, passing from West Berlin to East Berlin, and then up to Moscow. The journey would ideally unite East and West and sanction a more friendly diplomatic relationship between the two Blocs. The mere idea that a group of cyclists could pass through the Berlin Wall, resulting in the opening, albeit temporary, of the border with the Federal Republic of Germany, made Honecker's government shudder. The SED opposed the initiative, but Gorbachev was determined to carry out his project. At that point, the East Berlin Politburo pointed out that the possible opening of the border a few months after the famous Ronald Reagan 'Mr Gorbachev, tear down this Wall!' speech, in which the US President emphatically asked the Soviet leader to remove the Iron Curtain symbol, would give the world the impression of a certain subordination of the USSR to the American president. Gorbachev thought the East Germans might be right. Further organisational problems in involving the professional cycling clubs dealt the final blow to the idea, but the seed of a true opening between the two Germanys had been planted.

162

At the end of the 1980s, the East German government was cornered by an increasingly disastrous economic situation; the gross domestic product per capita was 40 per cent lower than that of the West Germans, and it became increasingly difficult to repay loans from non-socialist foreign countries. GDR President Erich Honecker had even tried to open up to Western markets but with inadequate results. At that time, one of the most pressing problems for the majority of the population engaging in so-called 'mass sport' was the chronic lack of sportswear, especially running shoes. Despite the noble intentions of the SED to invite people to run, hardly anyone could find suitable equipment in East German shops. In the archives of the DTSB, we can find hundreds of letters from angry citizens complaining about the scarcity of these consumer goods, a sign that the problem was very serious.[243] Strange as it may seem for a dictatorial state, East German citizens actually had the opportunity to protest to the authorities about any aspect of social life, through a communication mechanism known as *Eingabe*. The government took those grievances very seriously as they provided a realistic picture of the social situation and could help prevent any discontent on the part of the population. Whether the government's responses were satisfactory (or not) depended on several variables: the nature of the problem, the applicant's name, the tone of the letter, and the clerk dealing with the problem. Regarding the annoying 'shoe problem', very often there was nothing to be done. This lack of equipment had consequences for many younger athletes, discouraging them from pursuing their sports passion.[244]

---

243 Mike Dennis, Jonathan Grix, *Sport Under Communism – Behind the East German Miracle*, Palgrave Macmillan, 2012.
244 Ibid.

Meanwhile, the wonderful sports miracle machine was also starting to jam. Towards the end of the 80s, the talent recruitment system was undergoing a crisis that concerned the availability of the main 'ingredient': children. A slight decrease in births, and the fact that many parents (increasingly suspicious of the circulation of strange substances inside gyms) prevented their children from attending sports centres, had led the DTSB to consider the hypothesis of cutting, by a few years, the recruitment age. The Federation, however, did not have the power to take this decision, which belonged to the Ministry of Education, chaired by Margot Honecker. The GDR President's wife got in the way, claiming the right for all children to grow up in a natural environment appropriate to their age, at least until the completion of primary school. This dispute between the two structures created a reduction in the number of students enrolling in sports schools; there is no doubt that, if the Wall had not fallen in 1989, within a few years, the various sports delegations would have had to deal with a serious problem of talent scouting.

The end was near.

In an attempt to revamp a solid image of their system, and try to rekindle some patriotic enthusiasm, the German Olympic Committee dared put forward the candidacy of the city of Leipzig to host the 2004 Olympics, knowing that they would never have been able to financially support the project. The fall of the Wall shortly afterwards, and with it the entire East German state apparatus, spared them an embarrassing admission of bluffing.[245]

The Hungarian government's decision, in the summer of 1989, to open the border with Austria caused a massive exodus of East German citizens to the Federal Republic. On 9 November, the removal of the last barrier between East and

---

245 Barbara Cole, *The East Germany Sports System: Image and Reality*, University of Texas, 2001.

West, the infamous *Berliner Mauer*, resulted in the sudden demise of the socialist regime of the GDR and the gradual dismantling of the most complex, organised and efficient sports structure the world has ever seen.

8

MERITS AND HYPOCRISIES

WHAT WE have seen so far leads to an unambiguous conclusion about the practice of state-sponsored doping in East Germany and the complicity of politicians, managers and coaches, albeit with various levels of involvement: they have been proven to exist, beyond any reasonable doubt, by numerous testimonies and documents. We have also seen that the recruitment system for children from a very young age was one of the most efficient and sophisticated in the world, thanks to huge investment by the East German government.

In light of impeccable scientific and organisational competence, and a phenomenal commitment on the part of the athletes, in this chapter we will try to analyse their victories from a different point of view: the purely meritorious one. It will be an attempt to assume the role of the devil's advocate, to explore the possibility, both in a materialistic and ethical sense, that some of the medals won by the East German athletes could have actually been achieved exclusively thanks to their efforts; i.e. that some medals could in fact be made of pure gold and free from any chemical contamination. In addition, we will explore the issue of West German sports officials' negligence in setting up a proper doping trial, despite the evidence, and the corresponding relentlessness applied exclusively to GDR executives and athletes.

As a matter of fact, all the GDR athletes' victories certainly derive from a long and demanding personal journey made up of hard work, deprivation and intense training, which lasted for many years. It would be intriguing, if not strictly necessary, to know if among those athletes who won national and international accolades there were clean medal winners.

The documents and medical records found by Werner Franke and Brigitte Berendonk leave little room for doubt about the fact that a large number of athletes took drugs (either intentionally or unintentionally), but it is also true that the lists and archive documents are not exhaustive, i.e. there are many athletes whose activities cannot be linked to doping for certain. In addition to a certain documentary incompleteness, it must also be considered that in recent times some academics have begun to question the actual value of the *Stasi* reports. In particular, Professor Hermann Weber, a distinguished German historian[246], pointed to the fact that the notorious organisation often used so-called *Inoffizielle Mitarbeiter*[247], unofficial informers who didn't actually belong to the security forces; they were just ordinary citizens who didn't even receive any form of special training.[248] They were usually recruited 'on the go' and asked to spy and pass on information of some interest regarding family members or work colleagues, in exchange for some benefits. Some people did it voluntarily, while others were pushed or blackmailed. When the Berlin Wall fell, and it became possible to access the secret archives of the Ministry of Security, the names of these informants were exposed: betrayals were revealed, many families found themselves in conflict, long-standing friendships ended. Some people, despite the treachery, decided to forgive. In any case, IMs were non-professionals who jotted down and reported

---

246 He served as Professor of History at Mannheim University; he has been described as 'the man who knew everything about the German Democratic Republic' (*Die Welt*, 5 January 2015).

247 There were about 189,000! The term *Geheimer Informator* (secret informer) was in use until 1968.

248 *Mehr Stasi-Spitzel als angenommen*, Focus Online, 10 March 2008.

simple phrases, unusual behaviour and gossip that could, in their judgement, be useful to their controllers. Very often, they did a rough job. In fact, certain words could be misinterpreted or the spies themselves, in an attempt to appear efficient and useful, or because they might have resentments of some kind towards the people under surveillance, could have reported the events in an inaccurate or deliberately altered way.[249] Hermann Weber therefore warns that it would be wrong to carry out research and draw conclusions utilising exclusively the *Stasi* archives, because on more than one occasion they have revealed a distorted aspect of reality.

In order to achieve an accurate as possible reconstruction of the GDR sports system, in addition to the documents (after assessing their reliability), we should always consider the testimonies of the athletes and the people involved in that system. This has only been done to a certain extent. Journalist Frank Mertens, for example, reported the case of Dr Gertrud Fröhner, a sports doctor, whose name appeared in the archives of the *Ministerium* as an advocate of state-sponsored doping, but who was later exonerated by the testimonies of numerous athletes.[250] The doctor had indeed prescribed steroids, but only to a legally acceptable extent and limited only to the recovery of injuries in young gymnasts, and not aimed at improving their performance.[251]

Discus thrower Wolfgang Schmidt, a former world record holder, found out that he had been under surveillance

249 Hermann Weber, *'Asymmetric' bei der Erforschimg des Kommunismus und der DDR-Geschichte? Probleme mit Archivalien, dem Forschungsstand imd bei den Wertungen,'* Aus Politik und Zeitgeschichte. [Beilage zur Wochenzeitung Das Parlament], B26/27, 20 June 1997.

250 Frank Mertens, *'Leipziger Arztin weist Anschuldigungen von sich: Sporthistoriker Spitzer wirft Dr. Frohner Mittaterschaft vor,'* Leipziger Volkszeitung, 15 October 1997.

251 Robert Hartmann, *Glaubwurdiger Inhalt in Verraterischer Schrift,* Suddeutscher Zeitung, May 1998.

by the *Stasi* for many years, since he tried to defect. He was even arrested and sentenced to 18 months in prison. His file contains 2,000 pages! The documents reveal that, because he was a subversive, the secret police started rumours about him: they actually spread the word that Schmidt was a *Stasi* agent in order to isolate him from other athletes.[252] The fact that gossip, hearsay and false accusations were at all possible in East Germany, even coming from the *Stasi* itself, contributed to creating a degree of ambiguity around certain events and people's lives.

In the competitive arena, the situation of the well-known jumper and sprinter Heike Drechsler caused a sensation. The athlete had been accused for years of being a *Stasi* agent, an IM. Drechsler has admitted receiving performance-enhancing drugs without her knowledge, but has always denied being on the payroll of the Ministry of Security. Finally, in 2018, an investigation by researcher Helmut Müller-Enbergs established that Drechsler's name was actually listed in the archives as VIM (*Vorlauf-IM*), i.e. a potential informant, but she was never actually recruited. This inaccuracy has caused confusion and unfair accusations against the athlete from Jena.[253]

Hermann Weber also points out that only a small fraction of East German athletes (300 sportsmen and sportswomen out of a potential pool of 90,000 for the 1980s decade alone) had actually agreed to testify at the *Dopingprozess*; most of them were therefore never heard and we know nothing about their experiences.

British historian Mary Fulbrook has dealt with cases similar to that of Dr Fröhner, concluding that several athletes' reputations and careers were destroyed in an instant, once there was even the slightest link between the *Stasi* and

---

252 Grit Hartmann, *Goldkinder*, Forum Verlag Leipzig, 1998.

253 *Drechsler recruits expert to clear her name of Stasi link*, France24, 24 October 2018.

them.[254] The author does not deny the dramatic testimonies of the doping trial, but she affirms that in many cases, people became victims of witch hunts; in fact, there were numerous prominent positions available within the technical, medical and sports apparatuses of various bodies, such as universities, clubs and federations, which once belonged to East Germany, and that now appealed to people from the Western academic world. Following the trial, many East German executives were in fact fired and replaced by people from the West.

To give further credit to the thesis that in Germany, during the unification process, there was a risk of a one-size-fits-all approach, it is worth mentioning Ulrike Tauber's testimony. A gold and silver medallist at the Montréal Olympics, the athlete, while admitting to having received prohibited substances without her knowledge when she was a child, committed herself to a passionate defence of the category of coaches, stating that not all were the same and that many of them, in addition to being very well prepared, had refused to administer doping substances to their swimmers.[255] We saw some of these examples in Chapter 6.

Even people clearly implicated in the state-sponsored doping programme confessed their involvement but defended the athletes. Thomas Köhler, a former luger and DTSB vice president, admitted that while doping was widespread, some older athletes who knew about it blatantly refused to take drugs. He mentions lugers Ute Rührold, Margit Schumann and Eva-Maria Wernicke, who always declined doping because of the fear of gaining weight: they eventually won medals at the Olympic Games and the World Cup.[256]

254 Mary Fulbrook, *Anatomy of a Dictatorship: Inside the GDR, 1949–1989*. New York: Oxford University Press, 1995.

255 Christopher Keil, '*Das ist jetzt nur ein Teil der Wahrheit*,' Suddeutsche Zeitung, 19 August 1997.

256 *Ex-DDR-Sportfunktionär bestätigt flächendeckendes Doping*, Der Spiegel, 14 September 2010.

The allegations that doping was universally pervasive in East Germany are challenged by the testimonies of numerous athletes who have declared that they had never seen it happening. Of course, they could have lied, but many of them are people who have never won anything, so they would have nothing to hide or lose in admitting to having used steroids. In addition to them, there are athletes who have never been associated with doping, who won a lot and achieved Olympic glory, and were engaged in a type of sport, such as gymnastics or skating, which requires such high levels of technical skill and talent that it cannot be affected by drug use (see in this regard Manfred Höppner's documents mentioned in Chapter 1). For example, the East German athlete with the most medals at the Munich Olympics was gymnast Karen Janz, certainly a less well-known name than the swimming or athletics stars; she excelled in specialities where grace, strength and coordination are the result of innate talent and hard training, so it can reasonably be assumed that drugs would have been of no help, except possibly when recovering from injuries.

Moreover, the name of this gymnast does not appear in any *Stasi* document, as well as the names of hundreds of other athletes.[257]

Another competitor whose name was never associated with doping is Roland Matthes, a four-time Olympic champion widely recognised by friends and adversaries as one of the best backstroke swimmers of all time. Young Roland started swimming at the age of 11 under the watchful eye of Marlies Grohe, a coach known for her firm stance against doping, a moral position which probably cost her her career. Matthes became a champion before doping was imposed by law, showing he could dominate international races naturally;

---

257 Dieter Wales, Wolfgang Gitter, *'Milestones in the 30 Years History of the GDR: The Successful Seventies'*, Sports in the GDR, N.4, 10 October 1979.

the sport authorities recognised this and, at the insistence of his coach, left him alone.[258]

One of East Germany's top athletes and, perhaps, the one who found most fame and fortune, Katarina Witt, is another good example of how to excel in sport and also achieve considerable media recognition – she appeared on the cover of numerous Western magazines, including *Playboy* – without resorting to doping substances. On the surface, nothing that the skater was able to express on the ice rink, that is style, harmony and charm, seemed to be the result of a pharmaceutical programme. Witt's name has never appeared in any medical or *Stasi* records, despite her being one of the most surveilled people in the history of the GDR. The skater was in fact constantly spied on; given her growing international fame, the East German authorities feared that she might escape abroad. One of her skating colleagues, Ingo Steuer, was an alleged *Stasi* informant.[259] The dossiers on the athlete contained hundreds of pages about her, with infinitesimal details about her private life, but no notes ever referred to doping.[260]

So why do we also include athletes who did not dope, like Katarina Witt, Roland Matthes or Karen Janz ? Is it reasonable to assume their achievements were exclusively the result of hard work? Some researchers claim many documents have been destroyed and that some athletes may have doped and gotten away with it. However, in respect of these athletes, there is no claim or proof that any such files ever existed.

British scholars Mike Dennis and Jonathan Grix, for their part, promote the concept that doping, although widespread,

---

258 Karin Helmstaedt, *Swimming against the current*, The Whig-Standard, 5 May 2005.

259 https://www.faz.net/aktuell/sport/wintersport/eiskunstlauf-steuer-informierte-stasi-ueber-katarina-witt-1302155.html

260 *Germany skating coach Ingo Steuer tarnished by Stasi past*, The Guardian, 15 February 2010.

could not be the only discriminating factor: 'Oral-Turinabol was no magic blue pill, as performance-enhancing drugs had to be adjusted to individual training plans.'[261] Manfred Ewald's organisational ability in creating a sophisticated sports talent recruitment network has to be, to some extent, recognised. Dr Sigurd Hanke, a former athlete himself, is convinced that doping alone couldn't have been responsible for the GDR athletes' successes: 'I think there would have been good results even without doping. Not only was the recruitment system effective, but also the conditions we had as athletes were excellent: training conditions, food supply, adaptation of school lessons around training, physiotherapy, technology, and medical care.'[262]

In light of the testimonies and the academic considerations we have just seen, it could be assumed that, at least in some cases, the involvement of athletes and managers in doping was not active, and that further screening of the real collective responsibilities of an entire ruling class is necessary. The generic assumption that all the GDR athletes were (unknowingly or knowingly) cheaters and that they won thanks to chemistry should be seriously reconsidered and challenged.

Another interesting topic we should investigate further is the common acceptance of the distorted idea of East Germany's 'exclusive rights' on doping in the 1970–90 period. Doping has been exploited since 1990 as a weapon with which to discredit the GDR's achievements, yet most Western Bloc countries made extensive use of it. None of them have ever been subjected to the same level of political and judicial treatment.[263] Texan researcher Dr Barbara Cole makes an argument on the obsessive accusations by the West German

261 Mike Dennis, Jonathan Grix, *Sport Under Communism – Behind the East German Miracle*, Palgrave Macmillan, 2012.

262 Correspondence with the author.

263 Mike Dennis, Jonathan Grix, *Sport Under Communism – Behind the East German Miracle*, Palgrave Macmillan, 2012.

elite towards East German executives. According to Dr Cole, the assumption that GDR athletes had obtained their victories only thanks to doping (while other nations, such as West Germany, were almost immune to it) was artfully exaggerated for two reasons: revenge and dissimulation of their athletes' pharmaceutical habits.[264] It looks like the *Dopingprozess* represented an opportunity for historical revenge for the West Germans: after so many defeats and humiliations suffered in the stadia around the world, the time had come to retaliate. In a poll that appeared in the East German newspaper *Neues Deutschland*, the majority of Germans in the former GDR believed that the trial had more to do with a 'delayed revenge' rather than with a real determination to search for truth, and that it was not acceptable that only East Germany had hit the dock. In fact, even certain members of the Western press seemed to be on the same wavelength: the prestigious newspaper *Frankfurter Allgemeine Zeitung* argued that the *Dopingprozess* was essentially political and that it focused, on purpose, exclusively on the only aspect in which the former GDR shone: sport.[265]

In an article in the *Neues Deutschland*, Werner Franke himself was accused of adopting double standards. When the 5,000m Olympic champion, (ex-West) German Dieter Baumann, tested positive for nandrolone in 1999, Franke came to his rescue, explaining that, under certain circumstances, some steroids can originate naturally in the body. The defence did not hold up because the amount found in Baumann's blood was exaggeratedly high. The athlete, who pleaded innocent, suggested that someone had tricked him by inserting the steroid into his toothpaste; eventually, he was banned for two years.

---

264 Barbara Cole, *The East Germany Sports System: Image and Reality*, University of Texas, 2001.
265 Ibid.

Regardless of Baumann's case, it is certainly surprising to see such support from a researcher who accused an entire system of having abused precisely the same substance for years.[266]

The excessive relentlessness of the accusations against East Germany would also have served to remove the suspicions of doping that have hovered for years over some sports associations in West Germany, subsequently united Germany. In fact, numerous testimonies reveal the use of anabolic steroids by athletes from many nations participating in sport events. To remain in the German sphere alone, Helmut Digel, former president of the West Germany Sports Association, admitted that many of their athletes used doping during the 1970s and 80s. Some of them, such as weightlifter Ralph Reichenbach and heptathlete Birgit Dressel, even died due to a wrong dosage.[267] In an interview given to *Der Spiegel*, Dr Manfred Steinbach admitted that in the 70s he experimented with some substances based on steroids on underage athletes from West Germany. His candid justification for that obscene practice leaves one puzzled: 'It was just a scientific investigation, done at a time when anabolic steroids were not used in sports and were not illegal.'[268] The German magazine stresses that up to 1990, as many as 120 West German athletes had returned positive doping tests. In 1977, the chairman of the Sport Parliamentary Commission, Wolfgang Schäuble, denounced the passive and indolent approach of the various associations in the fight against doping and said that athletes, even then, were making some use of it.[269] Harm Beyer, director of the West German Swimming

266 Ulrike John, *Ist diese Leichtathletik noch zu rechtfertigen?*, Neues Deutschland, November 1999.

267 Andrea Schuelke, *Umsont Gestorben*, Deutschlandfunk, April 2017.

268 *Schicksalstunde des Sports*, Der Spiegel, December 1990.

269 J. Braun, *Very nice, the enemies are gone! – Coming to terms with GDR sports since 1989/90*, Historical Social Research, 2007.

Federation, confirms this information. Beyer admitted that he was an advocate of administering steroids to underage girls, although this procedure required parental consent. During his tenure, from 1977 to 1987, it has been claimed that numerous swimmers were instructed in the use of doping; among these, Nicole Haase and Jutta Kalweit.[270] Further confirmation of West Germany's interest in trying to optimise the use of anabolic steroids on athletes comes with the recruitment of the well-known Dr Hartmut Riedel, one of the greatest doping experts, in the laboratories of Paderborn University. Indeed, Riedel, who managed to escape from East Germany in 1987, quickly found a job in the 'mentally open' West Germany, managing a research centre for the use of doping substances.[271]

Former gymnast and vice president of the DOSB (the German Olympic Committee), as well as a member of parliament, Eberhard Gienger, also admitted to having voluntarily taken anabolic steroids for some period of his career.[272] In 1998, during the broadcast of *Sportschau*, a popular TV sports programme produced by the ARD channel, swimmers Chris-Carol Bremer and Mark Warnecke admitted on live television that 'in Germany, in the swimming discipline, doping is systematic and ubiquitous'.[273]

During the discussion in parliament regarding a law on compensation for doping victims, in 2002, Gustav Schur (cycling legend and member of parliament) pointed out that every year the German pharmaceutical industry produces about six tons of steroids, of which only 600kg (about 10 per cent) are used for therapeutic reasons. At the end of his

---

270 Mike Dennis and Jonathan Grix, *Sport Under Communism – Behind the East German Miracle*, Palgrave Macmillan, 2012.

271 Ibid.

272 *Eberhard Gienger: Habe Anabolika genommen*, Frankfurter Allgemeine Zeitung, May 2006.

273 Michael Muller, *Ganz vorn Schwimmen die Schlucker und Fixer*, Neues Deutschland, 20 October 1998.

speech, Schur wondered, not without rhetoric: 'Where does the rest go?'[274]

The 'hub' for prohibited substances was located at Freiburg University, a centre of excellence for sports medicine. West Germany had its own doping guru there: Professor Armin Klümper. The Freiburg doctor had been in contact with thousands of West German athletes for many years, including football players, and he was primarily responsible for administering performance-enhancing drugs.[275]

Discus thrower Alwin Wagner, and sprinters Birgit Hamann and Manfred Ommer, accused Klümper of being one of the largest doping providers in the world. Among his 'customers' there were also football clubs: the players of VfB Stuttgart and SC Freiburg, in the period 1979–80, took substantial quantities of Megagrisevit, a drug similar to Oral-Turinabol and which contained steroids.[276] Klümper was formally investigated in May 1984, but at the time there was an outcry by numerous sportsmen; some of them even started a fundraising campaign and collected millions of marks to help him face the court costs. Klümper eventually appeared like a victim of an injustice: his trial ended with a fine of 160,000 marks for money laundering – the doping allegations were forgotten.[277] In the 1990s, a new investigation was launched into Klümper but the doctor had already left Germany, having moved to South Africa.[278]

---

274 Horst Röder's website, http://www.sport-ddr-roeder.de, 29 January 2002.

275 J. Aumüller, J. Kelnberger, K. Ott e T. Zick, *Medizin für Millionen*, Suddeutsche Zeitung, April 2015.

276 Ibid.

277 Ibid.

278 Barbara Bürer and Nils Klawitter, *Seit 1990 schmückt sich der Westen mit den Sportlern aus DDR-Produktion. Ihre Schöpfer stehen nun vor Gericht*, Die Zeit, March 1998.

Even after Klümper's disappearance, his colleagues in Freiburg continued to care for German sportsmen throughout the 1990s, until the outbreak of the Team Telekom scandal, the cycling team whose riders were accused of taking concoctions based on orciprenaline and caffeine; among them, Tour de France winners Jan Ullrich and Bjarne Riis. The investigation into the doctors' illegal activities was eventually shelved and only in 2015 was it released to the public.[279]

Despite the assistance of the medical centre in Freiburg, the problem with some Western athletes was that doping, although widespread, was sometimes taken freely, with dosages often left to improvisation and without medical supervision: it was this that had perhaps led to the deaths of Dressele and Reichenbach. From this point of view, in East Germany there was a much more advanced level of experimentation and, paradoxically, a safer and more efficient method of distribution to the athletes (in the short term, at least).

In 2013, a report by some German researchers revealed that West Germany's athletes were methodically doped with government patronage from 1950 to (at least) the 1990s. The study was led by Dr Giselher Spitzer and carried out at Berlin's Humboldt University on behalf of the German Olympic Sports Confederation (DOSB). According to the report, the Federal Institute of Sport Science (BISp) financed experiments with performance-enhancing substances such as anabolic steroids, testosterone and oestrogen. The study claims that young boys and girls were also doped; they were not supposed to be given anabolic steroids because the long-term effects were unknown, but this limitation didn't stop the perpetrators.[280] Dr Spitzer's report contains

---

279 Detlef Hacke, *From Festina to Team Telekom/Team T-Mobile – Doping Scandals in Cycling*, Der Spiegel, found at www.uni-freiburg.de.
280 The Associated Press, *West Germany systematically doped athletes*, USA Today, 13 August 2013.

many revelations related to different competitions, but the names of the people involved have been concealed for legal reasons. There was a lot more to find out, but some sport federations refused access to their archives and the most relevant documents are now covered by a 30-year secrecy rule. It is evident that such a lengthy period serves the purpose of protecting a very dark secret and the reputations of very prominent people.

As many researchers have already reported in countless books and magazines, sports doping was also widespread overseas. Discussing this aspect in detail is out of the scope of this book, but here I would like to refer to a few significant episodes. As we have seen previously, anabolic steroids were in use in the 1960s. Former American discus thrower Jay Sylvester, winner of a silver medal in Munich 1972, after embarking on a career as a professor of physical education at Brigham University, said he carried out a survey on the use of steroids among athletes during the Bavarian Olympics. The result was that 68 per cent admitted to using them, testifying to the fact that there was already a certain spread of illicit drugs among the athletes of the time.[281] Sylvester says he saw athletes from different countries exchange pills of various kinds within the Olympic village, illustrating a certain transversal 'pharmaceutical camaraderie' and the acceptance of an established practice. In 1973, hammer thrower Hal Connolly produced a particularly eloquent sworn testimony before a US Senate Committee reporting that most of the American team members attending the 1968 Olympics had so many scars and holes in their backsides that it was difficult to find a free space to give them an injection.[282]

---

281 Terry Todd, *Anabolic Steroid: The Gremlins of Sport*, Journal of Sport History, 14, n.1, Spring, 1987.

282 Doug Gilbert, *The Miracle Machine*, Coward, McCann & Geoghegan, New York, 1980.

At the Montréal Olympics in 1976, a rather interesting case, which says a lot about doping and political dynamics, happened behind closed doors in the basement of the Olympic stadium. After winning the gold medal, discus thrower Malcolm Wilkins forgot to undertake a drug test. GDR top sport boss Manfred Ewald was present and revealed this episode in his autobiography: he proposed not to insist about Wilkins as he thought that reporting Wilkins's disappearance would have spoiled the friendly atmosphere of the event. The incredible thing is that if Wilkins had been disqualified, the gold medal would have gone to Wolfgang Schmidt, an East German! Seemingly, Ewald considered building a good diplomatic network more important than gold, on that occasion.[283]

In 2003, Dr Wade Exum, in charge of doping controls in the USA, confessed that in 1988 as many as 19 American athletes were granted permission to participate in the Seoul Games, despite the fact that they had tested positive in pre-Olympic tests.[284] Just a year later, before a US Senate Committee chaired by Joe Biden, sprinter Diane Williams admitted that she had received drugs such as Anavar and Dianabol from her coach.[285]

At some point, even American athletics legend Carl Lewis pointed out that the spread of doping in the United States was worse than in East Germany and that the world of sport was losing more and more credibility because of it.[286]

The above accounts constitute just a very small example; pending further data or confessions, we can certainly say that

283 Manfred Ewald, Ich War Der Sport, Elephanten Press, 1994.

284 www.nytimes.com/2003/04/17/sports/olympics-anti-doping-official-says-us-covered-up.html.

285 Lucas Aykroyd, *Health consequences of PEDs continue to plague ex-East German athletes*, Global Sport Matters, 7 November 2019.

286 *Lewis on the attack again*, Last Lap, Track and Field News, February 2000.

doping was not for the exclusive use and consumption of the GDR, but that it was also widespread in other countries, and that the unidirectional fury towards East Germany alone turns out to be quite hypocritical. Furthermore, united Germany has gradually absorbed laboratories, athletes, facilities, sports professionals and training techniques from the former East Germany. It would be useful to know what exactly of the East German experience has been assimilated. Even double Olympic javelin champion Ruth Fuchs, one of those athletes who took banned substances,[287] pointed out the great hypocrisy of the doping process due to the fact that certain pharmaceutical substances, although widespread all over the world, seem to have been used only in East Germany.[288]

State hypocrisy, however, found its consecration when hundreds of former East German athletes were 'absorbed' into the united German national team, after reunification. It would seem that, from the exact moment the two Germanys came together, all the shadows of doping suddenly disappeared. For example, swimmer Dagmar Hase, after being born and raised in the East, won most of her Olympic medals in the post-Wall era, so in a period commonly accepted as 'above suspicion', i.e. no longer subject to the state-sponsored doping regime; her victories are consequently considered clean. It is curious to note how German sports institutions attacked Hase for her past in the GDR, but then gladly accepted her to compete for united Germany. The same fate befell other swimmers such as Heike Friedrich and Daniela Hunger.[289] It would seem that, for every athlete who competed for both East and united Germany, there were two levels of judgement:

---

287 W. Franke: *'Die Täter sind die Ärzte' Athletinnen Fuchs, Otto und Enke wehren sich*, Frankfurter Allgemeine Zeitung, 9 April 1994.

288 Ruth Fuchs, *Die DDR, das Doping und die Pharisaer*, Neue Deutschland, January 1998.

289 *Die Doping-Lüge: Kristin Otto und andere überführt*, Berliner Zeitung, April 1994.

a severe one, to be applied before 1990, and a more flexible and accommodating one, post reunification. Hypocrisy of the highest order in action.

In this regard, shot putter Astrid Kumbernuss often complained about journalists' inquisitive questions because of her Eastern past, even though almost all of her victories took place after 1990. The athlete has always been a supporter of the GDR training system and thinks it was a pity that it was dismantled.[290]

The multiple swimming champion Franziska Van Almsick, despite having grown up in East Berlin, and having gone through all the stages of the typical youth sports preparation path (from the KJS schools to the *Spartakiade*), began to compete internationally only after the fall of the Wall. Hers is the most striking case of an athlete from the East who has found consecration and flawless glory with united Germany, Van Almsick has always openly criticised the lack of will of sports to fight doping.[291]

In short, many athletes from East Germany continued to excel many years after the fall of the socialist regime. There can only be two possibilities: either doping had disappeared (or in any case it wasn't really that influential in terms of results and performances), or its application continued, and was kept under wraps, even after 1990. As often happens, things are never black and white, and the truth lies in a large grey area, where a combination of the two options is the most likely eventuality, including that some GDR athletes never doped. Certainly, the axiom 'East Germans doped before 1990 and cleaned up after 1990' seems contradictory, superficial and very convenient for the various sports federations of united Germany. After the reunification, and therefore in a period

---

290 Jurgen Holz, *Uns wird ein Stempel aufgedruckt*, Neues Deutschland, October 1998.

291 https://www.espn.com/oly/summer00/news/2000/0914/744546. html

accepted – in theory, at least – as exempt from a doping system, the number of former East German athletes who contributed to the victories at the Olympics is enormous, certainly difficult to explain for those who advocated the theory that Eastern athletes won only thanks to doping. At the Albertville 1992 Games, where the united team of Germany unsurprisingly topped the medal table, 80 per cent of the wins were achieved by former GDR athletes, whilst in Barcelona the figure was almost 60 per cent. Still four years later, in Lillehammer, it was 60 per cent, and in Atlanta, 50 per cent. At the Nagano Winter Games, in 1998, 40 per cent of the German medals were won by athletes coming from East Germany.[292] Ten years after Seoul 1988, the children of socialism were still wandering around, obstinately successful, like ghosts of the past in the stadia around the world. These were athletes who grew up in the ranks of the KJS and in East Germany's sports clubs, going through training methods supervised by the GDR doctors. It is certainly grotesque that while on the one hand an entire nation was demonised, on the other, no time was wasted in incorporating elements of that system into the apparatuses of the new great united Germany. As we have already said: hypocrisy. To put it in the words of researcher Barbara Cole: 'The most compelling finding to emerge from the research of this system is that the image of sports in the GDR, both before and after *Die Wende*, has never been reflective of reality. One illusion has merely replaced another.'[293]

The grey area we mentioned above is fuzzy and difficult to identify, and it is not possible to draw general conclusions that fit all theories. The personal story of each athlete should be studied and evaluated separately because doping was indeed widespread but, as we have seen, there were quite a lot of

---

292 Barbara Cole, *The East Germany Sports System: Image and Reality*, University of Texas, 2001.
293 Ibid.

exceptions that depended on clubs, sport disciplines, years of activity, athletes' fame, personal coaches and how zealous IM spies and *Stasi* agents were. I think legendary swimmer Roland Matthes summarises well most athletes' mood: 'What bothers me is that people take it so easy and say that the GDR was leader at competitive sport because there was doping. This is black and white painting. This saves you the trouble of looking more closely. If you look at how the GDR sports science dealt with swimming, for example, there was a lot more to it: training methods, technical analysis, performance analysis, and so on.'[294]

We can certainly say that it would be unfair to deem a medal undeserved, if the athlete who won it didn't know or suspect anything about the state doping practices; especially if they were injected with drugs that didn't even benefit them. My inclination is to consider the victories of those athletes who did not know they had taken drugs morally valid; they appear to be, anyway, more ethically acceptable than those achieved by athletes who have consciously doped themselves. On the other hand, the defeated opponents rightly complain and ask for compensation. The opinion of the writer is that both the ones who were doped without their knowledge and those who finished behind them should be on the same podium step.

Both should be considered, at least morally, winners. From this point of view, I fully share the appeal by *Swimming World* magazine: 'Let the record stand – alongside every footnote necessary to make sport an honest place for future generations while treating victims on all sides with the dignity and recognition that they deserve.'[295]

---

294 Grit Hartmann, *Goldkinder*, Forum Verlag Leipzig, 1998.

295 Craig Lord, *GDR 30 Years On: The Day In 1989 The Berlin Wall Came Tumbling Down On Doping Regime*, Swimming World Magazine, 9 November 2019.

The stunned executives of the major international sports bodies should emerge from the dusty cloud of their bureaucratic formalities, scrape off the 'eight-year limit' rule, and have the political courage to do some sports justice, retroactively assigning *ex aequo* the medals to those who came behind the East German athletes. The fact that so many years have passed is irrelevant: justice, at least an ideal one, should always prevail. It would only be fair to give due recognition to those who deserve it, hoping that it does not arrive too late and be dedicated to their memory.

9

HELPING THE VICTIMS

ONE OF the outcomes of the *Dopingprozess*, which ended in July 2000, was that it legitimised for many athletes the status of 'victim of doping'. Once the sentences were pronounced, it was time for the former GDR sportsmen and sportswomen to join forces and seek compensation. In 2005, after a few years of meetings, studies and evaluations, about 200 former athletes decided to unite, with the assistance of lawyer Michael Lehner, to negotiate some form of reparation with the German Olympic Committee (DOSB), i.e. the sports' governing body that inherited functions and managers from the homologous association in the German Democratic Republic.[296]

Actually, in 2002, the *Bundestag* had decided to allocate, on its own initiative, a one-off compensation payment of 10,500 euro each for those athletes (about 300 people) who had managed to prove that they had suffered permanent damage to their health due to doping. The decision was positively welcome, but the figure decided by the German parliament was not sufficient to cover current and past medical expenses. Besides, moral damages were also included in that quota as a flat-rate. In addition to denouncing the DOSB, the former athletes decided to forward the same compensation request to Jenapharm (now absorbed by the multinational Schering),

---

296 Luke Harding, *Forgotten victims of East German doping take their battle to court*, The Guardian, 1 November 2005.

which had been responsible for the production of Oral-Turinabol and other drugs used by the East German doctors. The managing director, Isabelle Rothe, naturally denied any involvement by the company, explaining that Jenapharm was only the factory of the steroids (also used in therapeutic medicine) and that it had no direct responsibility for how these were used by the sports clubs and the athletes. Interestingly, the pharmaceutical giant certainly knew about the steroids' unpleasant side effects: 'If the treatment with anabolics is long-term, or at high dosages, real possibility for androgenic side effects exists. Skin conditions, such as acne, will develop; virilisation effects such as deepening of the voice, growth of facial hair, masculine habits, increased sexual appetite, and clitoral hypertrophy will all occur.'[297]

In December 2006, at the instigation of the Ministry of Sport, as many as 167 former athletes obtained the coveted compensation from the German Olympic Committee.[298] The parties agreed on a definitive payment of 9,250 euro for each athlete, who undertook not to seek further compensation in the future.

The payment made by the DOSB had the effect of inducing Jenapharm to consider an amicable settlement, without going through the courtroom; the pharmaceutical company reached an agreement with 184 former athletes for a final payment of 9,250 euro per person. The motivation for the compensation provided by Isabelle Rothe was explained as 'a social contribution to reduce the suffering of sick people'.[299] This was certainly an act of goodwill by the corporation,

---

297 Jenapharm paper, 1965, Reported in Craig Lord, *GDR 30 Years On: The Day In 1989 The Berlin Wall Came Tumbling Down On Doping Regime*, Swimming World Magazine, 9 November 2019.

298 *Compensation for Doped GDR Athletes*, Deutsche Welle, 13 December 2006.

299 DW Staff, *Drug Firm Jenapharm Compensates Doped Athletes*, Deutsche Welle, 21 December 2006.

the purpose of which was probably to rebuild its reputation; Rothe's action was completed with the generous allocation of a further 150,000 euro to be distributed to various associations involved in helping former athletes in difficulty or promoting anti-doping policies.

Unfortunately, state aid and compensation for some of the former athletes involved has been insufficient to cover all medical bills. Birgit Böse, director for a few years of a clinic for former GDR athletes (financed for a period by the German state but then closed), confirms: 'The funds had certainly given a hand to many of us, but they were not enough because certain diseases are chronic and severe and we had to put the money out of our own pocket to cure ourselves.' During her years as a consultant, Böse has helped more than 600 ex-colleagues whose lives have been ruined by doping, both financially and psychologically: 'One of the hardest things to accept, for anyone who has lived through that period, is seeing their former coaches still in business. People like Rainer Pottel (long jump), Gerhard Boettcher (discus), Maria Ritschel (javelin), Klaus Schneider (shot put) and Klaus Baarck (heptathlon) have confessed to having administered drugs for years, but they still work for various federations and often appear on television, perhaps to pontificate against doping.'[300] From Böse's words, a former athlete herself with numerous health problems ('My doctor told me that if I were a car, he would not hesitate to scrap me'[301]), it is clear that the German state was in a hurry to definitively cut the ties with the past, even at the cost of forgetting and forgiving certain behaviours.

At this point, considering the seriousness of the athletes' pathologies, these one-off payments seem more like a donation than concrete help to sort out their problems. After the 2005

---

300 Kyle James, *East Germany's doping programme casts long shadow over victims*, Deutsche Welle, 1 October 2010.

301 Kyle James, *The Quest for Gold Left Lives in Ruins*, Deutsche Welle, 29 September 2005.

reparations, they had to wait until 2016 before the German parliament decided to grant a further disbursement of 10.5 million euro to be divided among about 1,000 former athletes.

To act as a liaison between the victims and the aid fund, an association was created: the Doping-Opfer-Hilfe (DOH)[302], a Berlin-based consultancy centre that is responsible for informing and helping former GDR athletes get access to state compensation. This body, founded in 2013, was chaired until 2018 by former Dresden sprinter Ines Geipel (whose story we told in Chapter 5), with the assistance of numerous volunteers including Dr Werner Franke, lawyer Michael Lehner (president of the association since December 2018) and a group of psychologists willing to offer moral assistance to the victims. The support, coordination and data collection that Geipel has carried out in the last 20 years is truly commendable, especially if we consider that she has done it voluntarily. On the association's website there is plenty of information for all those who seek recognition as a 'victim of doping', an essential requirement for accessing any available form of financial support.[303]

'So far we have helped about 2,000 former athletes,' Geipel explains, 'but the funds allocated in 2016 are about to run out. We will have to fight for further financial recognition, also because in the meantime about 200 children have been added: children of people damaged by doping, and in turn suffering from various pathologies, such as skeletal deformations (especially in the limbs), hydrocephalus and mental problems.[304] The law does not currently recognise these "second generation victims". Sometimes, we can only offer psychological help; it's not much, but we think it's important

302 (Doping-Victim-Help) Headquarters: Robert-Havemann-Gesellschaft, Schliemann-straße 23, 10437 Berlin.

303 Correspondence with the author.

304 Ines Geipel, *Health Problems of Doping Victims of Former East Germany*, DOH website, 5 June 2017.

for them to know they're not alone. Lately, we have tried to calculate the number of deaths due to the consequences of doping: we have counted about 500, a figure higher than the number of people killed in the incidents around the Berlin Wall, in 40 years.'[305]

A long-term study on psychological and physical damage caused by doping is also underway. 'This project is based on a sample of 1,000 athletes from the former GDR,' explains Geipel, 'whose health is compared with that of the average population. The first results revealed that for former athletes the chance of developing a psychiatric illness, compared to a normal person, is 16 times higher.'[306]

As noted, many former athletes have permanent and debilitating conditions that prevent them from working. One of the aims of the association is to give legal support to these people to possibly get a state pension. So far, only rower Cornelia Reichhelm and canoeist Kerstin Spiegelberg have obtained one. The process for receiving the pension is particularly complex and Ines Geipel's consultancy centre tries to help applicants navigate the maze of German bureaucracy. The DOH centre is open to all German athletes, regardless of the type of sport, age or geographical origin. It is managed and self-financed by volunteers, with the help of the Federal Ministry of the Interior and through donations.

The association tries to offer individual advice, help with filling in an application for state contributions, and provide effective aid in the most difficult cases. Legal, medical and psychological assistance is also provided, as well as access to the Werner Franke archive, where former athletes can find information about themselves relating to their time in the GDR sports system. The initial purpose of the DOH

---

305 Holger   Zaumsegel,   *Mehr   Doping-Tote   als   Mauer-Opfer*, Ostthüringer Zeitung, 6 March 2018.

306 Ines Geipel, *Health Problems of Doping Victims of Former East Germany*, DOH website, 5 June 2017.

centre was to inform and assist in the period 2013–17, but the continuous increase in the number of people seeking help made it necessary to extend the service. Up to 2020, the centre has assisted around 2,000 former athletes. This figure gives a sense of how widespread post-doping illness is among sports competitors from the golden age of the GDR. And still many others could be added in the coming years. According to Ines Geipel, it will take another 30–40 years before the wounds heal completely: 'The 10,500 euro allocated, for some of them, is only symbolic; for instance, among the people we assist there is a former gymnast whose body was forced to remain short by drugs. Imagine something so unnatural: a body destined to grow but bottled in tiny dimensions. She is always in pain and in constant need of expensive care. It is clear that for some people the torment will never end.'[307]

Even today, there are former athletes who discover for the first time that they had been victims of a surreptitious doping system. Despite living with many health problems, some people have never turned to the authorities or to government funds. Why did it take so long before they decided to step forward? Ines Geipel has her own explanation: 'It must be said that many never thought of a direct link between their illnesses and their sport activity; some, on the other hand, were ashamed: it is not easy to talk about one's body reduced to a wreck. To overcome that sort of discomfort takes time.'[308]

In recent times, the centre has seen many former *Oberliga* football players. So far, there are 12 confirmed cases of footballers being victims of doping and they come from ten different teams. 'Many think that in football, given the modest results, doping was only minimally widespread,' underlines

---

307 Sven Geisler, '*Wenn du in diesem Land dopen willst, kannst du es problemlos*', Sachsische Zeitung, 4 June 2018.

308 Leaflet *Staatsdoping in der DDR*, Die Landesbeauftragte für Mecklenburg-Vorpommern für die Unterlagen des Staatssicherheitsdienstes der ehemaligen DDR, 2017.

Geipel, 'but the testimonies we have been gathering in recent months show the opposite. Some players of SG Dynamo Dresden and FC Carl Zeiss Jena told me about ampoules, syringes and pills of all kinds, circulating in the locker rooms, starting from the junior categories. Among the most common ailments, we found leukaemia, testicular cancer, alcoholism and depression. A very famous Dynamo player, whom I cannot name, came to see me the other day and told me that his life is almost over. He didn't want compensation, he just wanted to talk.'[309]

The DOH organisation is not the only centre in Germany that supports former athletes. Since 2016, the State Commissariat of Mecklenburg-Vorpommern on the Actions of the SED Dictatorship (LAMV) has been running an important reception and research centre for the study of long-term damage due to performance-enhancing drugs; they also try to provide valid psychological support.

As explained by the project coordinator, Dr Daniela Richter, the north-east state decided to set up the centre following numerous requests for help from its citizens, all former GDR athletes. 'After the ZERV investigations in the 90s, many of them discovered for the first time that they could be victims of that state-sponsored doping system and that they had taken certain substances without their knowledge; for them, the first point of reference was the authority of Mecklenburg-Vorpommern which, over time, developed a meeting point for these people. I think it is a model other states might follow.'[310]

The LAMV centre has so far helped 272 athletes (145 women, 127 men) from the areas of Schwerin, Rostock, Neubrandenburg and Stralsund. 'Many of those who come

309 Sven Geisler, *'Wenn du in diesem Land dopen willst, kannst du es problemlos'*, Sachsische Zeitung, 4 June 2018.
310 Correspondence with the author.

for help,' continues Richter, 'never talked about their condition to anyone; they feel misunderstood and even struggle to comprehend how their condition happened. Many of them suffered abuses of various kinds and also developed a certain dependence on the substances they were given [at a young age]. They often feel lonely and hopeless. We help them to regain their trust in themselves and also to obtain the necessary documents to access support funds; many of them have serious illnesses, especially fragile mental conditions, and we refer them to doctors who can best treat them. In addition to advice, we deal with scientific research and, above all, with public awareness, through conferences, lectures, interviews and distribution of informative material. This work of communication is necessary to help these people to achieve a degree of social acceptance of the traumas they suffered. The first step towards improving your condition is to recognise that you need help.'[311]

The work of Daniela Richter's team is really comprehensive; over time, they have informed most of the doctors in their area about the problem of state doping, so they can then encourage their former athlete patients to contact the LAMV centre. Of course, it is not possible, for confidentiality reasons, to reveal the names of the athletes involved, but Richter is nevertheless able to mention the cases that have particularly touched her. 'I have to say that they all have in common one thing: they lived through a very complex and highly controlled daily routine for years. Almost everyone had goals to achieve during training; if they did not reach them, they would be punished. A girl told me that one day they didn't let her go home just because she weighed a few grams more than she should. Their teenage lives were so absorbed in sports that they didn't have time to study other subjects. I have also noticed that many of them had problems with the development of their individual

---

311 Ibid.

personality. I was struck by the fact that many athletes never showed an interest in cultural or art areas, such as music, painting, dancing or singing; I also saw shortcomings in the psychosocial area typical of adolescents, such as dreaming, confronting others or having desires; all they have developed is a sense of self-discipline, due to excessive training combined with abuse of all kinds. Workouts were often a source of anxiety and demoralisation from verbal abuse; they feared not reaching goals or weighing too much – some told me they vomited in order to lose weight. Many reported episodes of psychological violence – they had to undress in front of everyone or go to the sauna fully dressed – but also of a sexual nature by doctors and coaches. In fact, almost all of them have undergone a process of objectification. In that system there was no room for the individual's development.'[312]

As was to be expected, many former athletes have now developed the idea that one must stay away from any kind of sport and all those who promote it. Growing up in a system where the main motto was, 'The state supported you, now the time has come to reciprocate with your success and your political loyalty', must have directed those young people towards a unique way of thinking. Trying to find alternatives to that world now is not an easy task: many of the former athletes are between the ages of 45 and 60, and they often experience situations of social disorientation. 'Most of the people who come to us are not primarily motivated by cash compensation,' underlines Daniela Richter, 'but by the need for human recognition. Many of them still haven't figured out how many substances they took; if they are sure about anabolic steroids, they do not know anything about other drugs used to reduce the side effects of Oral-Turinabol, analgesics to relieve pain or psycho drugs to increase concentration during competitions. The result of taking those long-lasting

---

312 Correspondence with the author.

pharmaceutical cocktails is the development of debilitating diseases; many suffer in fact from orthopaedic, gynaecological, oncology and mental problems.'[313]

The constructive work done in Mecklenburg-Vorpommern has recently inspired a similar commitment in Thuringia, where the *Landessportbund* (State Sports Association) has implemented a new system, a cooperation between the Thuringian State Chancellery and a doctors' network, to help former GDR athletes. Lawyer Anke Schiller-Mönch is the first person to contact for support. Initially, she would get only a couple of phone calls a week, but now she gets more; her team deals, at any one time, with 20 people a month. The *Landessportbund*'s policy is not to record any telephone number or name unless the caller agrees; they understand that in order to help these people, it is important to protect their privacy. 'Sometimes they just want to talk,' explains Schiller-Mönch. 'Sometimes they want us to go through the full process to get concrete help that normal doctors can't provide. When people report that they were competitive GDR athletes, this information often goes unnoticed. Some people are even insulted as fakers and hypochondriacs and can literally read the doctor's thoughts, saying: "What do you actually want? Back then you had privileges, travelled halfway around the world while we were locked up here; don't whine now!" There must be no such thing. There has to be awareness. Therefore – according to a suggestion from the Ministry of Social Affairs – from now on, the question of whether the patient was a competitive athlete in the former GDR should be included in medical history forms.'[314]

---

313 Correspondence with the author.

314 Pamphlet *Gemeinsam aus dem Schatten ins Licht, Dokumentation zum Symposium Doping und seine Folgen – Einsatz leistungssteigernder Mittel im Leistungssport der ehemaligen DDR und dessen Auswirkungen*, 24 August 2019, Bad Blankenburg.

For people with severe illness, Anke Schiller-Mönch's team tries to obtain a monthly state pension: this is very difficult to achieve, because they have to prove the link between ailments and doping. Unfortunately, this is a very lengthy process that involves the research of original documents which often are nowhere to be found. Besides, some institutions destroy them after 30 years. Some sort of simplification of the process is therefore needed. Schiller-Mönch thinks that under certain conditions, in order to speed up the process, the connection between the event and damage must be presumed, without asking for documents produced 40 or 50 years ago. Hopefully, the government will take this into account the next time it is going to provide financial help to the doping victims.

Certainly, more research into doping side effects would guarantee a more punctual response in identifying the connection between chemical substances, a sports career and illness. In a 2017 LAMV study, two psychiatrists from the research centre, Harald Freyberger and Jochen Burhmann, report that the severity of the long-term consequences for athletes subjected to doping, increases in line with the following factors: the duration of the intake of the substances, the dosage, the type of chemical compound, and the hardness of the workouts. In most of the cases examined, drugs were taken in pre-adolescence, for many years and in quantities ranging from 5 to 20mg per day. The cumulative effect must have been devastating. About 20 per cent of the athletes involved in the East German sports programmes developed diseases that affected their liver (with development into cancer), skin (acne and scars), intestines, hormonal control (menstrual disorders, infertility, erectile dysfunction), prostate (with the development of cancer), cardiovascular and skeletal systems – virtually all organs are involved, and many athletes have a combination of two or more ailments. Their quality of life today is very low. Many of them find it difficult to remember the events of their past due to the psychotropic effect of certain substances such as benzodiazepines and amphetamines. This memory loss makes it very difficult to reconstruct their experiences as young people.[315]

In the Stralsund and Schwerin psychotherapy clinics, the two psychiatrists take care of former athletes who have been diagnosed with mental disorders related to their doping experience. They receive personalised psychotherapy treatment through various sessions with a psychologist or with group therapies; in the most serious cases, the sessions are also accompanied by the use of antidepressant psychotropic drugs. No extra financial help is provided, but all treatments and medicines are free; this is greatly helping the former sportsmen and sportswomen who reside in those regions.[316]

As we have seen, the current health condition of many former athletes is particularly worrying, but it is certainly positive that the state now has structures to take care of them. It is, however, disheartening to see that in spite of such clear and dire consequences, athletes of all sports, all over the world, still decide to resort to doping in order to enhance their performances. Most of them will probably not suffer any short- or long-term health consequences, but by now they should all be aware of the fact that taking drugs is a very dangerous game of Russian roulette.

Ines Geipel is quite pessimistic about the future of the fight against doping because the temptations are now too many: 'We will never get out of it. People have to decide for themselves. I just hope that the athletes who decide to put their health at risk have taken out a good medical insurance policy, unless they wish to end up with a poor life like their

---

315 Leaflet *Staatsdoping in der DDR*, Die Landesbeauftragte für Mecklenburg-Vorpommern für die Unterlagen des Staatssicherheitsdienstes der ehemaligen DDR, 2017.

316 Ibid.

colleagues in the GDR.'[317]

In total, there are thought to be around 15,000 former athletes with health problems, both physiological and psychological. These people lived their lives in close contact with a world that, seen from outside, looked wonderful; it was considered a privilege to be accepted into one of the GDR sports clubs, and friends would usually look at those people with mixed feelings of respect and envy. For some of them there was even the chance to win a medal at an important international event, become famous, drive a blue Trabant, and maybe get an invitation to the futuristic Palast der Republik and shake hands with President Honecker. Was it worth it? Most likely not.

Now we know that glory and privileges in East Germany (but not exclusively there), came at too high a price and that many still pay, unjustly, for the consequences of choices that weren't entirely theirs. It is hoped that the powers that be might provide, once and for all, adequate financial and emotional support for the former 'diplomats in tracksuits', so they can find some deserved harmony, both spiritual and material, in the second part of their lives. After more than 30 years, these people are still aggravated by a regime that no longer exists (even the not-so-futuristic Palast der Republik has been demolished): a ghost country that continues to haunt its victims, decades later from beyond the grave. These were the heroes of socialism, the national icons and the world-famous sprinters who always crossed the finish line before the others: all of them now prisoners of a past they cannot forget and from which they cannot free themselves.

---

317 Sven Geisler, '*Wenn du in diesem Land dopen willst, kannst du es problemlos*', Sachsische Zeitung, 4 June 2018.

ADDENDUM

THE FADED HEROES

IN THE last year and a half, whilst this book was nearly ready for publication, we have witnessed one of the most controversial and inexplicable events revolving around a number of key people who managed the DOH centre. I have already mentioned a few pages back the fact that Ines Geipel was replaced by lawyer Michael Lehner as president of the organisation, at the end of 2018; in this section I will try to explain the reasons, sometimes surreal, that led to that change.

In the autumn of 2018, a group of people formed by Werner Franke, Henrich Misersky (both founders of the DOH centre), Gerhard Treutlein (pedagogue) and Claudia Lepping (journalist and former athlete) began to raise numerous doubts about the management of the organisation directed by Ines Geipel. In a dossier of about 60 pages, called 'Blackbox DOH', and presented to the *Bundestag* through the endorsement of some forces of the parliamentary left group, Franke and the others tried to challenge the facts that had emerged in 30 years of fighting against the East German doping system; they also criticised the way the DOH centre was being managed. In particular, Ines Geipel was accused of managing the funds a little too carelessly, giving 'victim status' to people who didn't deserve it.[318] The former sprinter was

---

318 Javier Caceres, *Bis das Blut schmerzt*, Suddeutsche Zeitung, 31 January 2019.

also accused of exaggerating and distorting certain events of her life in order to get government funding. Additionally, the report offered some considerations that border on the realm of historical revisionism, going so far as to declare that only a small proportion of the athletes were unaware of taking Oral-Turinabol pills, and that many of them, including minors, knew the origin of the substances they took. They also claimed it was not impossible for athletes to refuse certain substances, and said if they had wanted to leave the sports centres, they could have done so without suffering any consequence. The theory of forced doping was, in short, highly exaggerated, or at most a practice limited to a few isolated cases. Misersky even went so far as to argue that both the athletes and the parents were often aware of doping and that no one had chosen to give it up, except his daughter Antje![319] Misersky might be right, but it is worth remembering that he and his daughter were expelled from the national team precisely because of their dissent.

The group also questioned the 'second generation doping' assumption (i.e. the fact that there may be physical consequences for the athletes' children), and branded the proponents of that theory, from the Mecklenburg-Western Pomerania research centre, as 'dodgy'.[320]

In his dossier we read that 'internationally renowned scientists have studied the effects of doping for decades, excluding that their origin could be genetic or that they could be transferred from parent to child'. Again, Franke might be right but it would have been useful to include the names of those scientists in his report.[321]

---

319 Anno Hecker and Michael Reinsch, *Sind Opfer Versager?* Frankfurter Allgemeine Zeitung, 30 January 2019.

320 Javier Caceres, *Bis das Blut schmerzt*, Suddeutsche Zeitung, 31 January 2019.

321 Anno Hecker and Michael Reinsch, *Sind Opfer Versager?* Frankfurter Allgemeine Zeitung, 30 January 2019.

How is it possible that Werner Franke, the undisputed champion of the fight against state doping in the GDR, together with his wife Brigitte Berendonk, took such an initiative? Franke, in addition to being the founder of the DOH centre, was its manager for many years, working side by side with Ines Geipel and Michael Lehner. An attempt by Lehner to pacify Franke[322] was firmly rejected, as Franke replied that he did not want to have anything to do with people who lied for 30 years.[323] Harsh words, without an explanation.

The pivotal event that sparked the controversy was the request by Christian Schenk (decathlete, gold medallist at Seoul) to have access to the fund for doping victims, through the DOH. Schenk in his biography[324] had confessed that he took performance-enhancing drugs for a long time, knowingly, since the age of 20, but that he had never been informed about any side effects. The application, according to the 'Franke group', was an outrage to decency and had to be rejected: that is, Schenk should not have been entitled to any compensation. But, according to the criteria established by the DOH centre (in coordination with the German government), Schenk instead had every right to it. According to Ines Geipel, in the adolescent period of his life, Schenk had undergone state-sponsored doping without his knowledge: 'It is not that at the age of 18 there is a sort of cancellation of the abuses suffered during adolescence.'[325] Essentially, the fact that the decathlete later chose to take drugs voluntarily does not affect

---

322 Michael Lehner, 'Warum kündigen Sie den Doping-Opfern Ihre Loyalität auf?', Frankfurter Allgemeine Zeitung, 29 January 2019.

323 Anno Hecker and Michael Reinsch, Sind Opfer Versager? Frankfurter Allgemeine Zeitung, 30 January 2019.

324 C. Schenk, Riss: Mein Leben zwischen Hymne und Hölle, September 2018.

325 Anno Hecker and Michael Reinsch, Sind Opfer Versager? Frankfurter Allgemeine Zeitung, 30 January 2019.

his right to seek compensation for the period before he was 18. Physician and former athlete Dr Sigurd Hanke has a similar view. 'It is difficult to draw a clear line between victims and scammers but, in my opinion, victim status is given when due to emotional, political and legal (according to GDR law!) pressure, individual decision-making options were very limited or not available at all. In addition, minors were used without parental involvement, there was no comprehensive information that would have made an "informed consent" possible in the first place, and the drugs were secretly administered. [In Schenk's case] these conditions were probably mostly met. The mere fact that a state system establishes or even only allows practices towards its citizens, in which the citizens are viewed as "human material" in order to achieve wacky state goals, using its citizens practically as puppets, as soldiers or even slaves, is criminal and qualifies those affected as victims. The extent to which an individual opportunistically bows to the system in order to survive in it then recedes into the background.'[326]

The 'Schenk case' opened the Pandora's Box, exposing some alleged ambiguities of the DOH centre. According to the Blackbox report, Ines Geipel would have widened the access to funds a little too much, to practically anyone lamenting symptoms even vaguely related to doping, including people who had never been competitive athletes. Furthermore, through the research centre in Schwerin, Geipel would have obtained ad hoc scientific recognition for certain psychosomatic conditions, further increasing the number of people with access to the funds. The 'Franke group' therefore believed that a lot of public money was given too generously to people who should not have benefited from it, because their status as a victim of doping had in some cases been confirmed a little too easily. However, the request of the group

---

326 Correspondence with the author.

to the German parliament was not to cancel the aid given to the real victims but to review the criteria and parameters for allocating the funds. According to the accusers, the DOH centre had had a free hand for too long and enjoyed legislation that allowed it to use the money without accounting for how it was spent.[327] Following all the controversy that arose over those insinuations, Ines Geipel decided to resign from the post of president of the DOH. The former sprinter rejected the allegations, warning about the fact that the doping victims might be criminalized by this criticism.[328]

The theses contained in the Blackbox DOH dossier have sparked indignation among former athletes and journalists. In particular, the *Frankfurter Allgemeine Zeitung* lashed out at Franke, calling him 'full of himself' and commenting that if he were to persist with his absurd statements, he would risk tarnishing his own reputation.[329]

On 21 March 2019, a document questioning the management of funds by the DOH centre was presented to parliament. The petition bore the signatures of various left-wing representatives, with MP André Hahn being the first signatory. The document asked 43 questions about various aspects of the fund management by the organisation chaired by Ines Geipel, but also about the methods of ascertaining damage to victims.[330] The federal government replied on 3 May of the same year through a letter promulgated jointly by the Ministry of the Interior and the Ministry of Infrastructure. The government's response appeared to be

---

327 Gabriel Kords, *Neue Vorwürfe gegen Geipel und die DOH*, Nordkurier, 8 December 2018.

328 https://www.faz.net/aktuell/sport/sportpolitik/doping-opfer-hilfeverein-geipel-gibt-vorsitz-ab-15924221.html

329 Michael Reinsch, *Selbstgerechte Aufklärer*, Frankfurter Allgemeine Zeitung, 30 January 2019.

330 Deutscher Bundestag Drucksache 19/8636 19. Wahlperiode 21.03.2019

quite timely and exhaustive in all 43 points. Essentially, it renewed confidence in the DOH organisation and rejected any allegation by the applicants that the funds were managed irregularly or that there was an excess of victims benefiting from compensation. In addition, the *Bundestag* decided to increase the budget for the doping victims to ensure fund coverage until 31 December 2019.[331]

In the end, Ines Geipel's good work was confirmed by the government's response. As a further confirmation of her commitment, she was elected as honorary chairman of the DOH organization in November 2019.[332]

The response of the Merkel government therefore put an end to the unexpected theses presented in the Blackbox dossier, confirming the good work done by Ines Geipel and Michael Lehner. The real reason for those strange accusations will remain, at least for now, one of the many ambiguities of the long story told in this book.

The final and emblematic illustration of this strange story can be summarised in a photo (dated 15 August 2019) that portrays Michael Lehner tugging at former friend Werner Franke, trying to get him out of the room where the president of the DOH was organising a press conference.[333] After reading and evaluating the various aspects of this story, it really seems to be a psychodrama, with characters who in the space of a few weeks made a 180-degree turn from the ideas they had been advocating for more than 30 years.

This writer must confess that he has experienced feelings of great bewilderment. Even if Franke and his colleagues' accusations do not change by one iota the events

331 Deutscher Bundestag Drucksache 19/9830 19. Wahlperiode 3. 05. 2019

332 https://www.sueddeutsche.de/sport/sportpolitik-opferrente-als-ziel-1.4700015

333 *Eklat bei Pressekonferenz der Doping-Opfer-Hilfe*, Nordkurier, 15 August 2019.

and analyses of what happened in East Germany during the era of state-sponsored doping, they do create a certain intellectual embarrassment in the readers who try to extricate themselves from the convoluted narrative tangle of those events. Understanding and interpreting the reasons for such a doctrinal turnaround is, after all, analytical material that is beyond the scope of this book. Perhaps, the pure heroes, in the story told so far, never really existed, but there were simply people who, at the right moment, tried to seek justice, doing the right thing; the same people much later decided to change their position, perhaps following other benchmarks (fame?) that drifted away from the values they shared in the past. It can happen. People and circumstances change, but good deeds remain good deeds, no matter when or why they happened.

And right when I thought it was all over, I learned that hearings were scheduled in court, where Ines Geipel was seeking compensation from Henner Misersky for defamation: essentially, the former DOH advisory board member disputed certain statements Geipel had made in public and parts of her biography (including that she didn't stop competitive sport for political reasons but because of her poor performances). In November 2021, the Berlin Court decided that Misersky didn't defame Geipel. The former sprinter had to bear the costs of the legal dispute.[334]

The umpteenth chapter of a story that seems to have no end.

---

334 https://www.deutschlandfunk.de/ines-geipel-gerichtsverfahren-henner-misersky-102.html

APPENDIX I

DR RIEDEL'S LIST

List of athletes in Dr Riedel's thesis; claiming all of them received varying doses of anabolic steroids.[335]

Acronyms: HJ, high jump; SM, multidisciplinary sport; SP, sprint; SL, long jump; TJ, triple jump; PV, pole vault; DT, discus throw; PP, shot put; JT, javelin throw; HT, hammer throw

Ackermann, Rosemarie	HJ
Ader, Margit	SM
Auerswald, Ingrid	SP
Austel, Jens-Uwe	HJ
Bauer, Ulrich	SM
Beckmann, Simone	HJ
Beer, Ron	SL
Behmer, Anke	SM
Behmer, Bodo	TJ
Behrend, Ulf	SM
Behrendt, Kerstin	SP
Beilschmidt, Rolf	SL
Berg (Heyne), Almut	SL
Bergner, Thomas	PV
Beyer, Axel	SL, TJ

---

335 Modified from Brigitte Berendonk, *Doping. Von der Forschung zum Betrug*, Springer, 1991, p.181.

Beyer, Gisela	DT
Beyer, Monika	SL
Beyer, Ralf	PV
Beyer, Susanne	HJ
Beyer, Udo	PP
Bienias, Andrea	SL
Bienias, Gert	SL
Bohla, Michael	TJ
Boy-Garisch, Renate	PP
Brandt, Kerstin	SL
Briesenick, Hartmut	PP
Bringmann, Steffen	SP
Busch, Sabine	SP
Carlowitz, Jens	SP
Delonge, Andrea	HJ
Dittrich, Reiner	TJ
Dombrowski, Lutz	SL
Drechsler, Heike	SL, SP
Drehmel, Jörg	TJ
Dressler, Christian	HJ
Düring, Ute	HJ
Duwe, Heike	SL
Eckert, Bärbel	SP
Eckardt, Dirk	PV
Ehlert, Gaby	SL
Ehmcke, Petra	SL
Elbe, Jörg	TJ
Emmelmann, Frank	SP
Ernst, Petra	SL
Faltin, Elisabeth	HJ
Felke (Meier), Petra	JT
Fermumm, Heiko	TJ
Fiedler, Ellen	SP
Förster, Peter	HJ
Frank, Matthias	TJ, SL
Franke, Lutz	SL

Freimuth, Jörg	HJ
Freimuth, Uwe	SM
Fuchs, Sylvia	SL
Gamlin, Dirk	TJ
Geipel, Ines	SP
Geissler, Heidrun	SM
Gerstenberg, Detlef	HT
Giebe, Steffen	PV
Gladisch, Silke	SP
Göhr, Marlies	SP
Göhring, Romano	TJ
Gonschinska, Idriss	SP
Gora, Lothar	TJ
Grabe, Heike	HJ
Graf, Jens-P.	HJ
Grebenstein, Matthias	HJ
Gross, Axel	TJ
Grosshennig, Birgit	HJ, SL
Grosshennig, Ines	SL
Grossmann, Klaus	HJ
Grummt, Steffen	SM
Gründler, Andreas	PV
Günther, Olaf	SP
Günz, Gabriele	HJ
Gummel, Margitta	PP
Haber, Ralf	HT
Haberland, H.-Dieter	HJ
Hartung, Egbert	SM
Heidemann, Frank	SM
Heiland, Bernd	SL
Heimann, Sigrid	SL
Hellmann, Martina	DT
Heydrich, Angelika	SL
Hirschberg, Jens	HJ
Hirschke, Sylvia	HJ
Höhne, Mario,	TJ

Hölzel, Stefan	HJ
Hoffmann, Dieter	PP
Hohn, Uwe	JT
Holfert, Kerstin	HJ, SL
Hufnagel, Klaus	TJ
Hummel, Peter	SM
Huth, Bodo	HJ
Hyckel, Uwe	HJ
Jäckel, Frank	HJ
Jahn, Bettine	SP
Jentsch, Dietmar	SM
Jessat, Michael	HJ
John, Sabine	SM
Kanitz, Holger	SP
Kasten, Olaf	PV
Kazmierski, Detlef	HJ
Kempe, Antje	JT
Kertz, Sabine	SM
Kirst, Edgar	HJ
Kirst, Jutta	HJ
Kirst (Schmidt), Rita	HJ
Klein, Winfried	HJ
Knabe, Kerstin	SP
Knorscheidt, Helma	PP
Koch, Marita	SP
Koch, Mathias	SL
Kottke, Torsten	SL
Köhn, Christian	HJ
Konow, Manfred	SP
Kramss, Andreas	PV
Krieger, Heidi	PP
Krüger, Dieter	SM
Krumpolt, Joachim	PV
Kühn, Ute	HJ
Kühne, Wolfgang	SM
Külske, Frank-Peter	SL

Kurrat, Klaus-Dieter	SP
Lange, Joachim	JT
Lange, Uwe	SL
Langhammer, Uwe	PV
Laser, Christine	SM, SL
Lauterbach, Henry	HJ, SL
Lawrenz, Andre	SM
Lehmann, Marion	SL
Lemme, Armin	DT
Liegau, Ulrich	TJ
Liek, Frank	SL
Lindner, Wolfgang	SM
Löbe, Wolfgang	SP
Löffler, Eitel	SM
Lukowsky, Joachim	TJ, SM
Madetzky, Sylvia	PP, DT
Mai, Volker	DT, SL
Mangelow, Cornelia	SM
Maske, Frank	SL
Matzen, Doris	HJ
Meszynski, Irina	DT
Meuche, Günter	SL
Michel, Detlef	JT
Michel, Simone	PP
Moder, Mathias	HJ
Möbius, Sabine	SP, SM
Müller, Ines	PP, DT
Müller, Ralph	PV
Munkelt, Thomas	SP
Naggaltz, Ralf	SP
Natzmer, Holk	SL
Neubert, Ramona	SM
Neufeld, Renate	SP
Neumann, Burghard	PV
Nitzsche, Kristine	HJ, SM
Nowak, Frank	SL

Oschkenat, Andreas	SP
Oschkenat, Cornelia	SP
Pahling, Frank	TJ
Pappler, Petra	SL
Paschek, Frank	SL
Petersson, Jens	SM
Pfaff, Petra	SP
Pilz, Detlef	PV
Plöger, Erwin	SL
Pohlandt, Holger	SP
Pollak, Burglinde	SM
Potreck, Rositha	JT
Pottel Reiner	SM
Prenzler, Olaf	SP
Prystaw, Harald	SM
Pubanz, Udo	PV
Radtke, Helga	SL
Reichelt, Andre	SL
Reichelt, Marion	SM
Reinhardt, Wolfgang	PV
Rentz, Michael	SL
Rex, Thomas	TJ
Rieger, Peter	SL
Riecke, Hans-Ullrich	SM
Rodehau, Günter	HT
Rosenkrantz, Ulf	HJ
Rothenburg, Hans-J.	PP
Rübsam, Dagmar	SP
Rüdiger, Uwe	HJ
Rüdrich, Simone	DT, PP
Sachse, Jochen	SP
Sam, Andreas	HJ
Sandmann, Michael	HJ
Schäperkötter, J.-Peter	SM
Schauerhammer, Dietmar	SM
Schenk, Christian	SM

Schernikau, Bärbel	SL
Schima, Christina	SL
Schläger, H.-Peter	HJ
Schmuhl, Liane	PP
Schönlebe, Thomas	SP
Schröder, Manuela	HJ
Schröder, Matthias	TJ
Schröder, Thomas	SP
Schult, Jurgen	DT
Schulze, Cordula	PP
Schwabe, Henry	PV
Schwalbe, Marianne	SL
Seifert, Ulrich	SM
Siebert, Carsten	HJ
Siegl, Siegrun	SM
Slupianek, Ilona	PP
Sobotka, Jana	SM
Sommer, Marina	SL
Stark, Siegfried	SM
Stein, Ronald	TJ
Steuk, Roland	HT
Strobel, Katrin	JT
Sturzebecher, Udo	TJ
Techel, Toralf	PV
Thiele, Sybille	SM
Thorith, Detlev	TJ
Timmermann, Ulf	PP
Tischler, Heike	SM
Trampota, Wolfgang	HJ
Tröger, Anke	HJ
Ulbricht, Sigrid	SL
Voigt, Angela	SL
Voss, Torsten	SM
Walther, Gesine	SP
Warnemünde, Wolf.	DT
Wartenberg, Frank	SL

Weber, Axel	PV
Weigt, Britta	HJ
Weiss, Gerald	JT
Wendland, Eberhard	SM
Wessig, Gert	HJ
Wienick, Peter	PV
Wiese, Ronald	SM
Wodars, Frank	SL
Wolfram, Carsten	TJ
Wujak, Brigitte	SL
Wycisk, Heidemarie	SL
Zachert, Falk	SM
Zech, Petra	HJ
Zenk, H.-Joachim	SP
Zwanzig, Andreas	SL

APPENDIX II

STEROIDS FOR WOMEN

A non-exhaustive list of East German sportswomen and the average amount of anabolic steroids it is claimed they took each year.[336] The values take into account the regularly registered pills. According to Dr Hartmut Riedel's studies, the maximum recommended doses of Oral-Turinabol should not have exceeded 1,500mg for men and 1,000mg for women in one year. As can be seen from the list published below, these limits were often surpassed.

Acronyms: SM, multidisciplinary sport; SP, sprint; DT, discus throw; PP, shot put; JT, javelin throw.

Ines Müller-Reichenbach	3,680mg	PP
Irina Meszynski	3,190mg	DT
Helma Knorscheid	2,900mg	PP
Ilona Slupianek	2,615mg	PP
Heidi Krieger	2,590mg	PP
Silvia Madetzky	2,390mg	DT
Bärbel Wöckel-Eckert	1,670mg	SP
Bettine Jahn	1,560mg	SP
Cornelia Oschkenat	1,480mg	SP
Kersting Behrendt	1,474mg	SP
Marita Koch	1,460mg	SP
Margitta Gummel	1,450mg	PP

---

336 Brigitte Berendonk, *Doping. Von der Forschung zum Betrug*, Springer, 1991, p.211.

Marlies Göhr	1,405mg	SP
Anke Behmer-Vater	1,380mg	SM
Ingrid Auerswald	1,375mg	SP
Ramona Neubert	1,340mg	SM
Ines Geipel-Schmidt	1,291mg	SP
Gesine Walther	1,290mg	SP
Martina Hellmann-Opitz	1,255mg	DT
Sabine Möbius	1,230mg	SM
Dagmar Rüsbam	1,230mg	SP
Sabine Busch	1,230mg	SP
Petra Felke	1,185mg	JT

APPENDIX III

COURSE OF STUDY AT DHfK, LEIPZIG

Subject Semester (Lessons per week)								
	I	II	III	IV	V	VI	VII	VIII
Fundamentals of Marxism	2	3	4	4	3	3	2	4
Introduction to Logic	3							
Sport Pedagogy	2	2	2			3	5	
Sport Psychology	4	4					2	
Theory and History of PE					3			
Sport Politics						2		
Guide to Socialist Physical Culture						3	3	6
Mathematics and Cybernetics	3	2			2	2		

Fundamentals of Natural Sciences	6	3	3					
Sport Medicine	1				3	3	2	
Biomechanics				3			2	
Theory in Training	15	17	11	18	11	12	10	
Sport Practice			6	6	6	6	6	6
Sport Theory		5	5	5	5	5	5	5
Foreign Languages	2	2	1	2	2	1		

Modified from Gilbert, *The Miracle Machine*, Coward, McCann and Geoghegan, NY, 1980.

APPENDIX IV

ONE LAST THOUGHT

The East German athletes' autographs: symptom of a generation of sport legends vanished into thin air.

The author of this book considers himself a nerd and a collector. One of my regular activities is attending sci-fi and sport conventions; here I can meet and greet movie, television and sports stars. These brief but meaningful encounters allow me to chat to celebrities, take a selfie, and purchase their autographs. Regarding the latter, their value, and therefore the price, varies according to the degree of popularity of the personality in that particular period of their career; the autograph fee can also change over time. For example, remaining in the world of sport, the autograph of a footballer from the England team that won the World Cup in 1966 costs around £20–25; that of an eternal champion like Pelé, can reach £200. In short, there is a well-regulated market, complete with a price list and certificates of authenticity.

Some time ago, I happened to come across an autograph sales site in Germany. Among various stars of all sports, present and past, with prices that more or less corresponded to those of other dealers, there were many genuine autographs of athletes from the GDR. I was struck by the fact that the prices were very low. We are talking about £3–5 for very famous athletes who won tons of medals. I couldn't really explain that at first. I gave it some thought and I realised that, perhaps, the aura of negativity that pervaded these athletes, following the doping scandal, has kept sport enthusiasts away, causing the prices of this particular market to drop. Probably, collectors are not as interested in buying autographs of characters who are forever linked, in many ways unjustly, to unsportsmanlike conduct and to cheating.

Ultimately, even something as trivial as a signature on a photograph can become the emblem of a piece of history that many would like to forget.

INDEX

INDEX

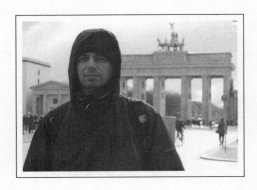

THE AUTHOR

Joseph Tudor was born in Sesto San Giovanni, Italy, in 1969, and currently lives in Essex (UK).

Truly passionate about sport and TV series, this publication is his first on a historical subject.

He has a BSc in geology and a BA in humanities, as well as a Post-Graduate Certificate of Education (PGCE). He has been teaching science and history since 2000.

In his free time, he plays oboe and French horn with the Clacton Concert Orchestra.

Also available at all good book stores

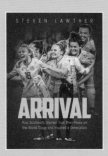

9781785318276

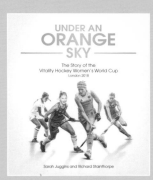

9781785314926

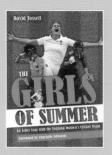

9781785311352

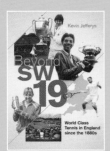

9781785317767

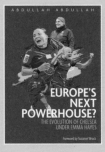

9781801500500

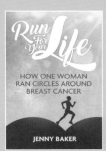

9781785312618

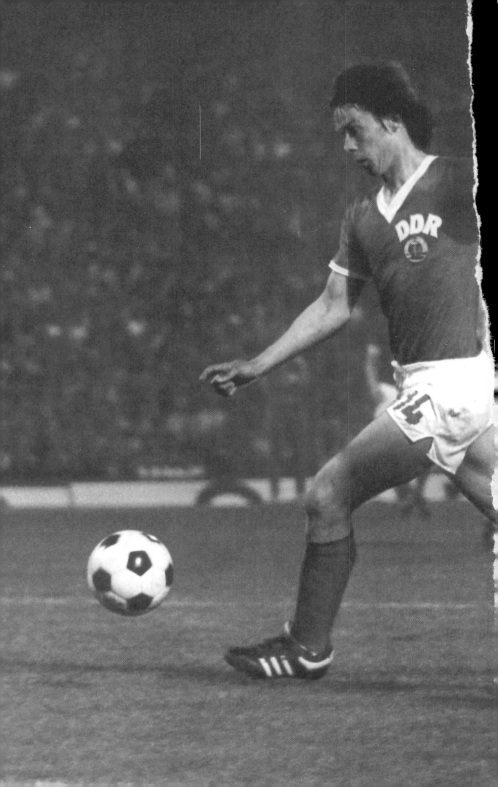